ELECTROCHEMICAL ANALYSER IMMUNOSENSOR DESIGN FOR DETECTION OF SWEAT CORTISOL MECHANISMS

ANKIT GUPTA

CONTENTS

LIST OF FIGURES

Chapter I

Introduction

1.1 Background and overview

The World Health Organization (WHO) has witnessed cardiovascular disease (CVD) as one of the leading cause of death globally and the mortality rate due to CVD has increased annually than any other cause in the developed and developing countries [1]. Their recent survey divulged that the CVDs take lives of 17.9 million people every year, 31 % of all global deaths. CVDs can be caused by a range of factors and disorders including high blood pressure, cholesterol, diabetes, obesity or overweight, smoking and stress [2]. Among these factors, psychosocial stress is reported to be a major cause for CVDs [3]. Suffering from stress is becoming a global issue and it affects the people's ability to take decision at work including police, soldiers in combat, athletes or anybody in emergency situation (Fig.1.1). There is growing evidence that stress is harmful to health as it alters the immune system leading increased propensity to infections.

Since the globalization and modern lifestyles influence genetic disorder and imbalances in protein concentration and human metabolism, which are major roots of diseases. These systems are deemed as pioneer technology for the improvement of both global healthcare and health disparities monitoring. The development of diagnostics tools is indeed for quantifying the specific biomarkers and of providing health informatics for superior treatment strategies. Non-invasive point-of-care (POC) monitoring devices will be helpful in such scenarios as they would aid rapid diagnosis and treatment of people suffering from stress [4, 5]. In particular, POC aim to replace centralized hospital based care systems with home based personal diagnostics to reduce healthcare costs and real time monitoring by providing non-invasive, factual analysis for accessing human performance [6, 7]. The demand for real-time healthcare monitoring devices is rapidly increasing due to the numerous benefits that this technology offers from social, scientific and financial perspectives.

Recently, miniaturized sensing devices have been explored for biomarker detection in order to decrease the probability of human error and the sample volume required. The obtained data can be used to evaluate health informatics in timely disease diagnostics. In this context, wearable sensor devices either supported on human body or piece of clothing can be exposed their prominence in health diagnostics at POC. These devices are described as autonomous and non-invasive systems that perform a specific monitoring of target analyte in physiological conditions and provide substantial observation, data storage and processing.

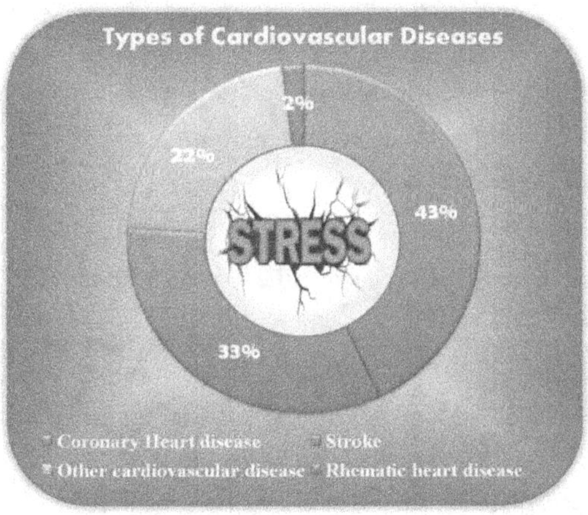

Fig. 1.1 Cause of cardiovascular diseases - a recent survey

1.2 Cortisol

Cortisol is a steroid hormone, recognized as a key molecule in the psychobiology of stress and related negative health outcomes. It is one of the important glucocorticoids (a family of steroid hormones) produced by adrenal glands. Cortisol is a small molecular weight (362.46 g/mol) hormone with the chemical formula of *(11α)-11,17,21-Trihydroxypregn-4-ene-3,20-dione*. Fig. 1.2 illustrates the chemical structure and the 3D arrangement of the cortisol.

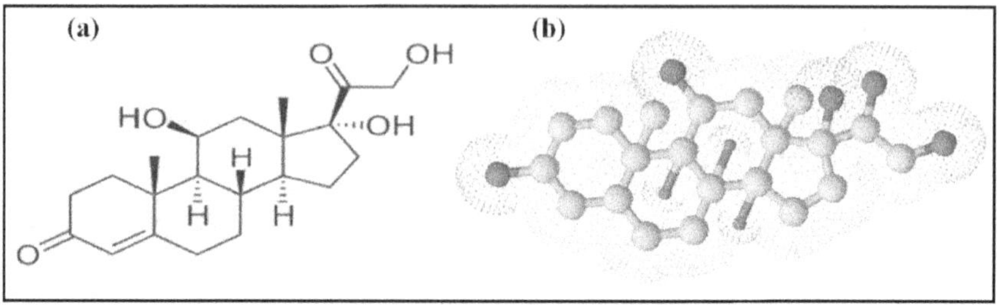

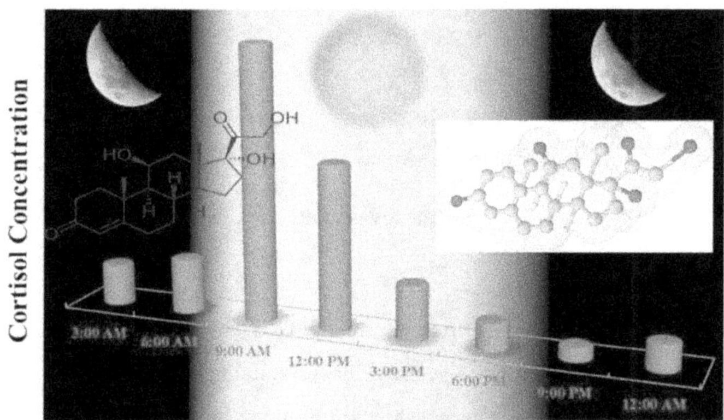

Fig. 1.2 Chemical structure of cortisol: (a) 2D and (b) 3D

Cortisol plays an important role in human physiology, the regulation of various physiological processes such as blood pressure, glucose levels and carbohydrate metabolism. It also plays a vital role in homeostasis of the cardiovascular, immune, renal, skeletal and endocrine system [8-10]. Cortisol levels fluctuation over a period of 24 hour cycle are called the circadian rhythm (Fig 1.3), highest during daybreak (30 min after awakening) and progressively lower by night [11]. Apart from the day-night cycle, several controllable factors can affect cortisol levels such as eating patterns and physical activity [12].

Fig. 1.3 The representative diurnal variation of cortisol levels over a 24 hour cycle

Abnormal increase in cortisol levels inhibits inflammation, depresses immune system, increases fatty and amino acid levels in blood. While excess cortisol levels have been shown to contribute to the development of Cushing's disease with the symptoms of obesity, fatigue and bone fragility [13], decreased cortisol levels lead to Addison's disease which is manifested by weight loss, fatigue, and darkening of skin folds and scars [14, 15]. Insufficient amounts of cortisol can cause nonspecific symptoms such as weight loss, low blood pressure, fatigue, muscle weakness and abdominal pain. The most dominating effect on cortisol variation comes from psychological/emotional stress, which is why cortisol is popularly called the "stress-hormone" [16, 17].

Increasing level of psychological stress due to the globalization, altered living style and struggle is becoming a serious concern in everyday schedule and life threatening diseases such as heart attack, depression and brain pain are the health challenges faced by the most developed countries. The potential causes of health disparity in everyday lifestyle are numerous. The precise and accurate detection of psychological stress is thus gaining consideration for personalized health monitoring and diagnostics [18, 19].

1.3 Secretion of cortisol

Cortisol is a hormone that is secreted from the adrenal glands located above the kidneys. Cortisol is the end product of the hypothalamic–pituitary–adrenal (HPA) axis, which is the main component of the human body's adaptive system to maintain regulated physiological processes under changing environmental factors. As the name suggests, the HPA axis is a complex signaling system among the hypothalamus in the brain, the pituitary glands and the adrenal glands [19, 20].

Fig. 1.4a presents a schematic of the HPA axis in which a typical response to an environmental trigger is initiated at the hypothalamus that releases a hormone called the CRH (corticotrophin releasing hormone) that travels to the pituitary glands. Specialized cells that work synergistically with the pituitary glands release ACTH (adrenocorticotrophic hormone) into the blood stream that travel to the adrenal cortex.

The adrenal cortex is responsible for increasing the production of cortisol. The produced cortisol then goes to participate in all the governing physiological processes. Since the adrenal glands have no visible innervation, it can be inferred that ACTH is the sole stimulant for initiating cortisol production. The adrenal glands do not store cortisol, but they are prevalent in the form of precursors.

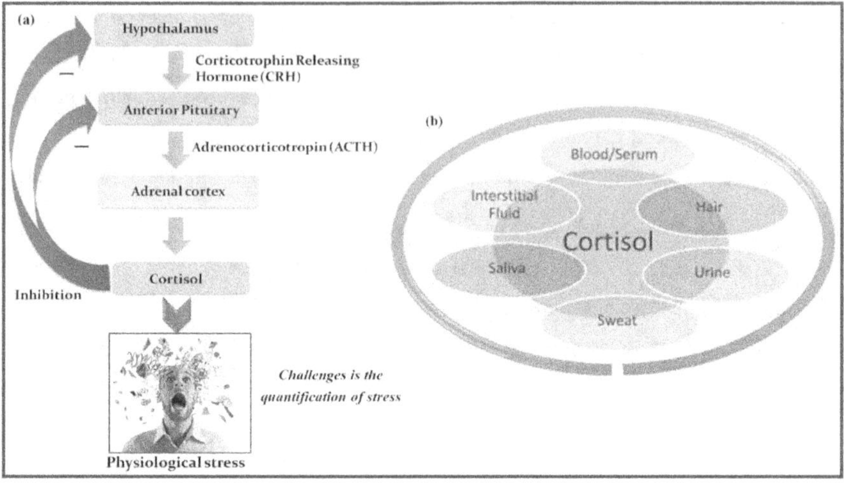

Fig. 1.4 (a) Cortisol secretion regulated by the HPA axis and (b) various bio-fluids used for cortisol evaluation

Cholesterol undergoes multiple catalyzed oxidation reactions to result in the formation of cortisol. This entire process takes place in a time space of few minutes. The HPA axis is a negative feedback system, where cortisol plays a critical role in the homeostasis of the HPA axis. Moderate homeostatic alterations in the HPA axis are beneficial for the physiological and the psychological development of the human body. The sustained and prolonged exposure to environmental triggers such as stress leads to abnormal levels of cortisol in the circulatory system [8].

1.4 Sources of sample

Secreted cortisol finds its way into the circulatory system and can be found in detectable quantities in several bio-fluids. In this section, an appraisal of the advantages and disadvantages of using various bio-fluids such as urine, blood, sweat, interstitial fluid (ISF) and saliva for the detection of cortisol is presented (Fig. 1.4b) [21].

1.4.1 Urine

Cortisol level in urine is measured over a day and is referred to as the 24 hrs urinary free cortisol (UFC) test. Only free cortisol, which is the active form of cortisol in the human body, is found in urine and is consequently a relevant biofluids for the detection of cortisol. The excretion of hormones, salts and other waste chemicals through urine is a diagnosing tool to locate and quantify the specific waste substances under normal function. Observation of drastic variation in concentrations of hormones such as cortisol can be used to diagnose irregularities in the adrenal function. Measurement of cortisol in urine usually requires the collection of all the urine generated over a 24 hrs time period. Normal range for cortisol in urine is 10–100 µg/24 hrs. A review of the reported literature for urinary cortisol assays has been presented by Brossaud et al. (2012).

Although, the 24 hrs urinary free cortisol test offered a means for a non-invasive, painless method of obtaining body fluid for cortisol measurement, it also caused several drawbacks with respect to convenience and reliability. Since the collection of the urine is spanned over a 24 hrs time period, sample collection becomes an inconvenient process where the patient needs to carry the special urine collection container all day long or has to remain confined to a location for the 24 hrs period. The container also needs to be stored under refrigeration from the time of collection till it is delivered to a diagnostic lab for testing. Also, several factors such as pregnancy and medication such as diuretics can alter the concentration of cortisol in urine making it a lesser reliable bio-fluids for cortisol detection. These several other factors have severely limited the use of urine in cases where patients are admitted to the hospital for long-term treatments. The requirement of 24 hrs sample collection has rendered urine unfit for real-time detection at POC [22].

1.4.2 Interstitial fluid (ISF)

ISF is an extra cellular fluid that surrounds the cells in the human body. In composition, it is similar to blood plasma. Metabolites and proteins move into ISF as they move from capillaries to cells. In general, small to moderate sized molecules including glucose, ethanol and cortisol, are found in ISF in similar proportion as in blood. Thus, periodic calibration using blood sampling is not required to obtain the concentration of these metabolites from ISF. The ISF is present just below the skin, but the low permeability of the epidermal keratinized layer (the stratum corneum) blocks the permeation of the fluid through the skin. However, obtaining ISF for the detection of a target biomarker could require an invasive approach as it is not readily accessible.

Several approaches have been reported in the literature to obtain ISF in a minimally invasive and painless process. Venugopal *et al.,* (2008) have reported the construction of an ISF harvesting system that utilizes a low-energy laser to create micropores in the stratum corneum (the uppermost layer of dead cells). The diameter of the micropores is approximately equal to that of a human hair. The micropores only penetrate the stratum corneum and hence, this procedure is essentially painless. ISF is drawn through these micropores continuously by the application of a small amount of vacuum pressure. Harvesting of ISF using this set-up is reported at a rate of 10 mL/h [23]. Coupled with an electrochemical detection system, Venugopal *et al.,* (2011) have reported the detection of cortisol using the same microporation set-up. Cortisol levels in ISF were found to be 3–4 times larger than that in saliva, which makes ISF attractive bio-fluids for the detection of cortisol. While this set-up may provide a means to access ISF for cortisol detection, the low harvesting rate (10 mL/h) would limit its applicability for obtaining instantaneous cortisol values in a POC setting [17].

Mukerjee *et al.,* have reported the design, fabrication and testing of a hollow microneedle array containing fluidic micro channels for the transdermal extraction of ISF from human skin [24]. Wang *et al.,* (2005) have also reported the fabrication of glass microneedles for ISF extraction for glucose monitoring. These approaches show promise for creating painless, minimally invasive methods for extraction of ISF. Microneedles based transdermal ISF extraction may find good application in wearable biosensing system, where there is a critical need to continuously sample body fluids such as ISF at a low sampling rate [25]. However, concerns regarding biocompatibility and biodegradation of the microneedles, protection from infection due to usage of needles and other sterility issues will need to be carefully addressed for successful implementation.

1.4.3 Hair

The use of hair as the biological sample for analysis and testing in forensic sciences, toxological science, doping control and clinical diagnostics has gained considerable attention over the last two decades [26]. Human hair grows at a predictable rate of approximately 1 cm/month. Cortisol is known to deposit in the shaft of the hair and the most proximal 1 cm segment of hair closest to the scalp approximates the last month's cortisol production and so on. The mechanism for the incorporation of cortisol into the hair shaft has been proposed by Bennett *et al.,* [26]. Cortisol is thought to enter hair primarily at the level of the medulla of the hair shaft via passive diffusion from blood. In this scenario hair cortisol would be hypothesized to reflect the integrated free cortisol fraction rather than the total cortisol concentration in serum.

One of the first studies to establish feasibility of using hair for cortisol detection was reported by Koren *et al.,* (2002) [27] using hair from wild hyraxes. Detection was performed using a modified salivary ELISA protocol. *Sauve et al.,* (2007) [28] reported the first study on human hair samples for cortisol detection and reported a reference range from 1.7 to 153.2 pg/mL. The obtained values were compared to those obtained from saliva, serum and 24-h urine. A positive correlation was identified only to that of 24-h urine, with no correlation to that of saliva or serum. Hair cortisol measurement surely provides a non-invasive method of obtaining a biological sample. Since the cortisol concentration in hair is hypothesized to represent long-term system exposure, it could be used as an indexing method to maintain a cortisol secretion calendar. From the various other reported studies [29-31] for cortisol detection from human hair, it is evident that cortisol values only for long-term exposure to factors such as stress can be obtained. The resolution of the data obtained is in the order of months, with very little clinical data available to support the correlation of hair cortisol levels to stress levels.

1.4.4 Blood

More than 90% of cortisol in blood is in an inactive state being bound to corticosteroid binding globulin (CBG) and serum albumin. Only 10% of the total cortisol is in a biologically active state to participate in cortisol initiated processes. Typically assays for measuring cortisol in blood involve measuring the total cortisol (bound+free) and then the active fraction, called the Cortisol Free Index (CFI) is deduced using Coolen's equation [32]. Blood sampling for cortisol detection has been the oldest form of bio-fluid sampling. The nominal value for cortisol in blood varies from 25 mg/dL (9 AM) to 2 mg/dL (midnight), which has many drawbacks and last choice of sampling fluid. Sampling blood requires attention from medical staff and specialized, sterile equipment with an ever-existing concern for infections. While cortisol is an unstable molecule at room temperature, its presence in plasma requires special handling and storage condition as it is considered a biohazard. Since sampling blood requires puncture of veins, a painful procedure, the stress experienced by patients prior to and during sampling may elevate cortisol levels [33]. Although the typical response time for cortisol spiking is 10-15 mins in humans, prior knowledge of veinpuncture can initiate the stress response induced cortisol spiking. Also, the costs associated with staff, equipment, handling and storage make the blood based assay a shunned option.

1.4.5 Saliva

Over the last few years, saliva has gained considerable attention as a bio-fluid for analysis and detection of cortisol concentrations. This has come about mainly due to the inherent advantages associated with saliva. First and foremost, a well-documented strong correlation exists between salivary and blood cortisol levels [34, 35]. Also, of high importance is the fact that cortisol in saliva exists entirely in the free state unlike in blood (90% bound), resulting in the detection of the relevant (biologically active) form of cortisol. This is mainly due to the filtering of the CBG and albumin bound cortisol during capillary exchange and other intracellular mechanisms at the salivary ducts. Harvesting samples for analysis is almost completely non-invasive with little or no discomfort to the specimen providing the sample [36]. The last few years has observed the establishment of standard operation procedures for collection of saliva, which has led to lesser variability in analyzed results. The samples can be harvested with minimum efforts that have facilitated patients to collect their own samples at home. The advantages associated with salivary techniques have led to saliva being on the limit of becoming the preferred source of body fluid for the detection of cortisol. Also, the ease of sample collection, handling and storage has heightened its prospects for applying in point-of-care sensors for real-time and continuous detection of cortisol.

However, there are certain aspects that may adversely affect the prospects of saliva based cortisol detection. Since only the active component of cortisol (free cortisol) is present in saliva, the concentration of cortisol is much lower than that of blood. Moreover, the room temperature instability of salivary cortisol possesses the problem of storage during on-site sample collection and processing. Also, the nominal values for cortisol in saliva during the diurnal cycle vary from 0.5 mg/dL to 0.05 mg/dL, which require high sensitivity assays with low detection limits for efficient detection of cortisol concentration in saliva. Deviation from the standard operating procedure for saliva collection can lead to erroneous results. Sometimes, the presence of blood due to oral lessons may lead to elevated levels of cortisol and cause erroneous results. Salivary cortisol assays have been reported in the literature extensively for characterizing the circadian rhythm [37], Cushing's syndrome [38], Addison's disease [39], adrenal abnormalities [40] and stress related disorders [41].

1.4.6 Sweat

Sweat is the body fluid that provides significant information about health for diagnostic purposes. Different proteins and metabolites contained in sweat help identify disease or infection and also provide information about general health status. Researchers are being done for real-time health monitoring using sweat to detect glucose, lactate or other electrolytes. But no biosensor system has been successfully developed to detect cortisol from real sweat. Development of a sensor system using sweat cortisol is a challenging process, as it requires extremely high sensitivity compared to other forms of cortisol [42]. Cortisol in sweat has been measured by Russell *et al.,* [43] with cortisol concentrations ranging from 141.7 ng/mL (daytime) to 8.16 ng/mL. Human sweat contains abundant information about a person's health status and thus is an excellent bio-fluid for non-invasive sensing [44]. For example, sodium, lactate, ammonium, and calcium levels in sweat are indicators of electrolyte imbalance [45] and cystic fibrosis (CF) [46], physical stress [47], osteoporosis [48], and bone mineral loss [49] and etc., Continuous detection of the above mentioned analytes is highly desired for optimal physiological balance. Sweat has also been used for monitoring a person's intoxication level [50] and signs of drug abuse [51], among other applications.

When compared to various bio-fluids, sweat is the most extensively evaluated non-invasive body fluid as it contains plethora of medical information for diagnosis. It is comparatively easier to stimulate, collect and analyze [52]. Sweat based monitoring overcomes many of the shortcomings related with blood based assays.

Different approaches have been applied to enhance the sensitivity and selectivity of cortisol in sweat. Nanomaterials like Zinc oxide have been used by R. D. Munje *et al.* to immobilize number of linker molecules for specific detection of cortisol [21]. However, the existing techniques have still not achieved enough sensitivity and specificity to detect sweat cortisol. Sweat is the next level tool that can be applied to develop POC cortisol sensor system which allows continuous monitoring of sweat compared to saliva or hair, to assist health treatment and diagnosis.

1.5 Detection of Cortisol: State of the art

Cortisol has been detected using various methods as shown in Fig. 1.5. Having studied the physiology of cortisol and evaluating the pros and cons of the different sources of bio-fluids for cortisol detection, this section provides a comprehensive overview of the various detection techniques for quantification of cortisol [52].

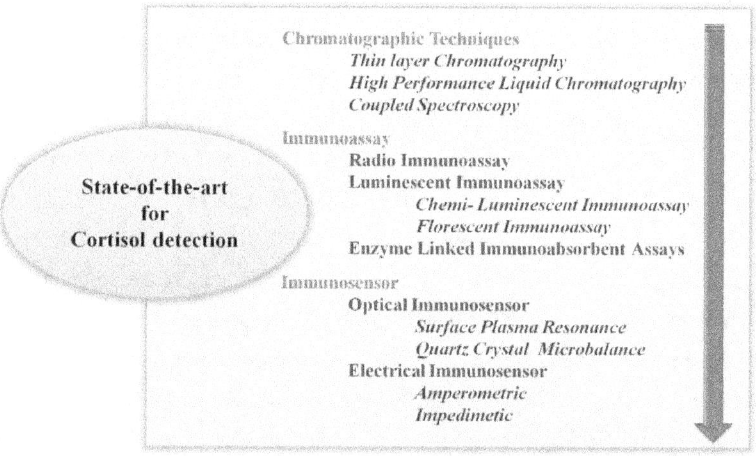

Fig. 1.5 State-of-the-art for cortisol detection

1.6 High Performance Liquid Chromatography (HPLC)

HPLC is the older and one of the first techniques to detect cortisol. HPLC is a chromatographic technique that used high pressure (50 to 350 bar) to separate a mixture of compounds using a process of mass transfer induced adsorption. While RIA was used to determine cortisol in serum, HPLC was used to determine cortisol concentrations in saliva. HPLC lacks the specificity that is required in measuring low concentrations, as the technique is severely affected by interference from co-eluting substances in the sample. HPLC also requires many pre-processing procedures such as solid-phase extraction [53, 54].

1.7 Immunoassays

Immunoassays are based on the ability of an antibody to recognize and selectively bind to an antigen, referred to as the analyte (Fig. 1.6). The high degree of selectivity and specificity of an antigen–antibody binding makes immunoassays the gold standard technique for the detection of presence and measurement of the concentration of the analyte of interest.

After successfully capturing the analyte, traditional process of immunoassays employ a label to detect the analyte. Enzymes, fluorescent tags and radioisotopes are some of the commonly used labels. Immunoassays may be performed in different configurations, depending on the analyte, label and detection technique. The primary classification of immunoassays is based on washing (heterogeneous) and no-washing (homogenous) of the sensing substrate after sample incubation. While homogenous immunoassays involve lesser assay steps, its application is limited by sensitivity and noise arising from nonspecific interactions. Heterogeneous immunoassays are further classified based on competitive/noncompetitive and labeled/unlabeled binding of the antigen to the antibody (Fig. 1.6). In a competitive immunoassay, the analyte of interest (unlabeled) competes with a known concentration of labeled analyte of the same kind. At the completion of the reaction, the concentration of the unbound, labeled analyte is measured, from which the concentration of the analyte of interest is deduced (Fig. 1.6a). Accordingly, in a noncompetitive immunoassay, only the analyte of interest is allowed to freely bind to the antibodies and a then the analyte is labeled to measure the concentration (Fig. 1.6b). To increase the sensitivity and selectivity of the immunoassay, a two-site or sandwich immunoassay is performed, where two a pair of antibodies are used, one for capturing the analyte and the other for detection (Fig. 1.6c).

Several transduction techniques have been developed to obtain measurable signal that is proportional to the concentration of the captured analyte and can be broadly classified as optical and electrical.

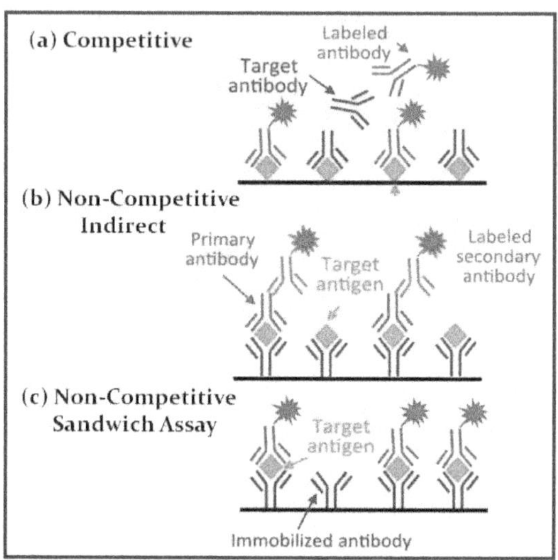

Fig. 1.6 Schematic illustration of various immunoassay techniques

1.7.1 Radioimmunoassay (RIA)

For the detection of cortisol, radioimmunoassay (RIA) which involves the use of radioisotopes as label was reported in the late 1970's [55-58]. Since the 1980's use of RIA has diminished due to the potential harmful effects of handling radioisotopes. The focus has shifted towards the use of labels with fluorescence property. The uses of fluorescent tags such as fluorescein isothiocyanate (FITC) [59], mixture of sulfuric acid and acetic acid [60] have been used as the label in cortisol immunoassays. A fluorescence detector is utilized to read the intensity of fluorescence, which is proportional to the concentration of the fluorescence labeled analyte.

1.7.2 Electrochemilumenescence immunoassay (ECLIA)

Another popular optical based immunoassay is the electrochemilumenescence immunoassay (ECLIA). ECLIA is based on the electro-generated chemilumenescing property of intermediates undergoing a highly exergonic reaction to produce an electronically excited state that emits light. ECLIA has developed into highly reliable immunoassay technique due to the high sensitivity and precise control over the electrochemical reaction. ECLIA has found application in many clinical studies for cortisol detection in human samples for Cushing's syndrome [61, 62], obesity [63], athletic disorders [64] and stress related disorders such as PTSD [65, 66].

1.7.3 Enzyme Linked Immunosorbent Assay (ELISA)

All the available labeled immunoassays, Enzyme Linked Immunosorbent Assay (ELISA) is the most sensitive, versatile and is today considered the gold standard in protein concentration determination. ELISA is typically performed in a sandwich format, where an enzymatic substrate is added to the secondary antibody to amplify the colorimetric or fluorescent signal, thereby providing a high sensitivity. Detection of cortisol using ELISA is used widely [67, 68] has often been the technique used to validate results obtained from newer techniques being developed for cortisol detection [69]. ELISA kits for detection of various analytes are commercially available now. While this method is the most widely used technique in research labs and industry, the method is limited by the need for large sample and reagent volumes and complexity arising from multiple assay steps and large incubation times. To overcome the tedious processes, cost and shortcomings of the assay performance, focus has shifted towards developing label-free immunosensing techniques with high sensitivity, lower detection limits and broader detection range [70]. One such technique that demonstrates label-free detection is based on Surface Plasma Resonance (SPR) [71].

1.7.4 Surface Plasma Resonance (SPR)

SPR works on the principle of oscillation of valence electrons in a conducting substrate irradiated with light. SPR is highly sensitive to adsorption of molecules onto the substrate, where the resonance curves shift to higher angles with adsorption of molecules onto the surface. SPR has shown promise as a method to quantitatively measure the capture of analyte on substrates coated with anti-bodies. The associated detection optics and electronic for SPR measurement can be reduced to miniaturized form factors and has hence attracted efforts to create point-of-care immunosensors [72]. More recently, detection of cortisol in saliva [73] and other biofluids using SPR has been reported in literature. On the same lines as SPR, another technique gaining ground for immunosensing is based on the resonance property of quartz crystal microbalance (QCM) [74-78].

1.8 Electrochemical sensors

Based on the electrical property being measured, electrochemical sensors can be classified as potentiometric, voltammetric and Impedimetic sensors. Potentiometric immunosensors passively measure the potential between two electrodes. The set-up consists of an electrode pair, where the potential on one electrode is maintained constant (reference) and the potential at the other electrode (immunoelectrode) is measured with respect to the reference electrode. The immunoelectrode usually uses electrodes that have been made ion selective. The measured potential can then be correlated to the concentration of the analyte directly from the Nernst equation. Potentiometric immunosensing is not a popular strategy due lack of sensitivity, accuracy, precision and stability [79]. This is due to a basic assumption that the measured potential accurately reflects the equilibrium position of an electrochemical reaction, which is often not the case. The interference arising from the sample matrix will supersede the signal arising the specific binding of an analyte.

Voltammetric techniques involve the application of a constant potential to the immunoelectrode surface and measuring the resulting steady state current generated by the electroactive redox species. It may be noted that the difference between voltammetry and amperommetry is trivial and confusion in literature is due to the introduction of scanning techniques in voltammetry, where the potential is help for a brief length of time (for current measurement) and then increased/decreased for further measurements. Voltammetric techniques can be described as a function of Voltage, Current and Time. Linear sweep voltammetry (LSV), the potential at the working electrode (immunoelectrode) is swept at a specific rate (volts/sec) from a lower potential to a higher potential and the current at each potential step is measured [80]. A variant to this technique, called cyclic voltammetry (CV) entails applying a triangle potential waveform from an initial value to a predetermined upper limit, where the direction of the sweep is reversed [81]. As the potential is swept back and forth, the current on the working electrode is observed. Analysis of the current response can be used to study the thermodynamics and kinetics of electron transfer at the electrode solution interface. Moreover it helps to study the kinetics and mechanism of solution chemical reactions initiated by the heterogeneous electron transfer. CV can also be described as an analytical tool by which information about the analyte can be obtained by measuring the current flowing on the working electrode that either oxidizes or reduces the analyte. The magnitude of this current is proportional to the concentration of the analyte in solution, which allows CV to be used in determination of the analyte concentration. The current at the working electrode (faradaic current) can be plotted as a function of time or since the potential is linearly related with time, as a function of voltage. The representation of the response in CV experiment is usually the current-potential curve, which is called "cyclic voltammogram" (Fig. 1.7).

As the potential is swept in the forward direction, a cathodic peak is observed. Reduction occurs in this positive scan and the current resulting from the reduction is called cathodic peak current. The potential value in this point is called as cathodic peak current potential. These representations of these terms are i_{pc} and E_{pc} respectively. Note that the reduction current is taken as positive as the cathodic sweep goes from left to right. At the switching potential the direction of the potential sweep is reversed. In the reverse scan, oxidation occurs and a peak resulting from the oxidation process is called anodic peak current. A negative anodic peak current is observed in the case of oxidation process. The representations for the anodic peak current and anodic peak potential are i_{pa} and E_{pa} respectively. A diagram of the electrochemical workstation (SP 50) and typical cyclic voltammogram is given in Fig 1.7(a & b) with a clear representation of the defined characteristics such as i_{pc}, E_{pa}, I_{pa} and E_{pa}.

Efforts are being made to develop wearable detection analytical devices to quantify stress and related abnormalities in environmental condition to gain useful information for timely diagnostics and treatment. Studies have linked cortisol levels with human stress and hence cortisol has emerged as a most potent biomarker for physiological stress detection [9, 82].

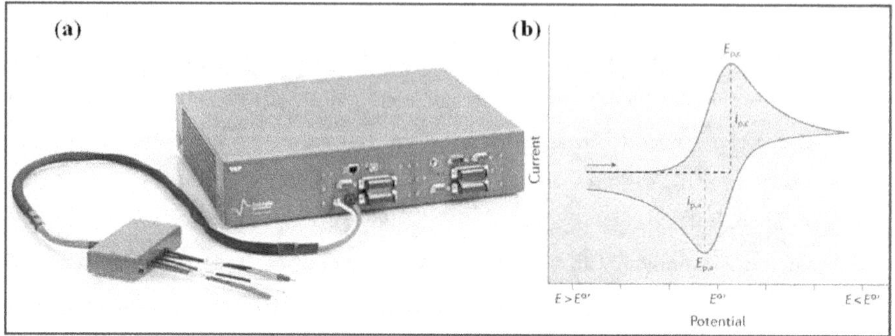

Fig 1.7 (a) Diagram of the electrochemical workstation and (b) typical cyclic voltammogram with defined characteristics

There has been growing interest in measurement of cortisol to establish whether cortisol variation can be used as a precursor to medically and psychologically relevant events such as stress, the most recent affliction being post-traumatic stress disorder (PTSD) [83, 84]. Since cortisol secretion is dependent on environmental and behavioral triggers, its measurement at POC has become imperative to understand behavioral patterns.

1.9 Electrochemical Immunosensing

Since the focus of this dissertation is on developing strategies for cortisol detection based on electrochemical immunosensing, this topic is discussed elaborately. Among the label-free technologies for detection in immunosensing, electrochemical immunosensing has emerged as the most promising alternative to optical detection.

Electrochemical immunosensing is based on the principle of measuring the changes in electrical properties of a conductive material due to the adsorption of an analyte on the surface functionalized with antibodies. The electrical change is attributed to the change in the concentration of the electro active redox species at the electrode proximity. The mature processing capability of the microelectronics industry has allowed building microelectrodes that provide high sensitivity and very low detection limits. The simplicity of electronic circuitry for electrochemical detection and cheap volume manufacturing has driven efforts to bring electrochemical immunosensing up to speed with other immunosensing techniques [75, 76]. The elementary requirement for an electrochemical immunosensor is a conductive substrate, which permits the immobilization of antibodies. Metals such as Au, Ag and Platinum and carbon electrodes intrinsically allow adsorption of antibodies, but the resulting binding is not robust and stable enough. To overcome this problem and to improve the electrochemical response, nanomaterials are employed as a linker molecule between the electrode surface and the antibodies. The choice of material is dependent upon the formation of bond with the conducting electrode surface and the presence of functional groups on the nanomaterials for covalent binding to antibodies [77].

Many strategies for sensing the immuno-reaction exist and is symbolized in Fig. 1.8. The traditional sandwich immunoassay may be utilized, in which, the secondary antibody is an antibody-enzyme conjugate, and the added enzyme substrate produces an electro active product that can be measured at the electrode surface (Fig. 1.8a). A simpler and efficient strategy, called the direct assay, involves measurement of the change in electro activity of the electrode due to the reduced electro active probes arising from the spatial blocking of the electrode surface area by the adsorption of the captured analyte (Fig. 1.8b). This technique may besimple, however sometimes lead to false positive results due to non-specific adsorption and hence effective chemical strategies need to be employed to non-specific adsorption [52, 78].

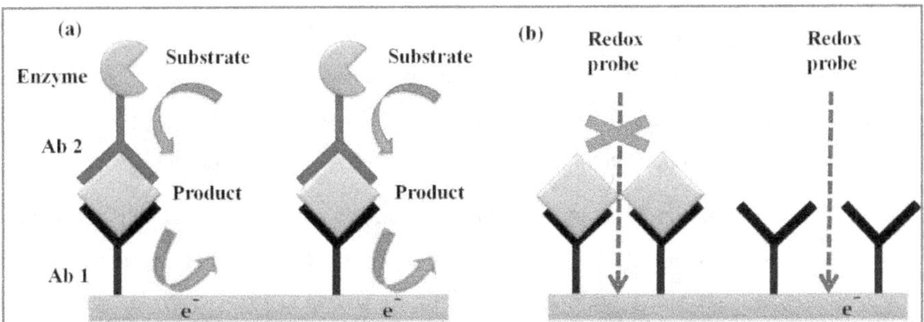

Fig. 1.8 Schematic of strategies used for electrochemical immunosensing

1.10 Why we need wearable sensors?

In recent years, there has been growing interest in the development of wearable biosensors, which would open up a revolutionary opportunity to monitor patients even in remote areas which is key for the development of modern healthcare [85, 86]. Wearable health monitoring technologies and devices are of great and continuous interest in clinical healthcare due to their ability to monitor physiological signals and to help maintain an optimal health status as well as assess the physical fitness of outpatients. To meet the special requirement of wearable sensors, the binder-free material with free-standing structure emerges which can effectively simplify the electrode preparation process and improve the electrochemical performance.

Imagine a world in which electronics are freed from their rigid, confining encapsulation, are closely integrated into the fiber of our daily lives and distributed throughout our ambient environment. This is impossible to do using conventional electronic circuits, which are limited by the maximum substrate size available for processing, substrate rigidity and fragility. Textiles represent an attractive medium for electronic integration as they have been a fundamental and transformational component of our everyday lives for hundreds of years. Smart textiles represent the drive to integrate new sensing functionalities into hitherto inaccessible surfaces and are a new step in the continuing evolution of textiles [87].

Smart textiles also known as electro or e-textiles fall into the category of intelligent materials that sense and respond to environmental stimuli. In contrast to smart textiles, functional textiles are materials to which a specific function is added by means of material, composition, construction, and/or finishing (e.g., *by applying additives or coatings*).

For smart fabrics, the targeted application plays a considerable role in the required conductivity of the conductive yarn. Some textile applications (e.g., lighting applications) may require considerable current and low ohmic (high conductivity) wires are preferred. Certain sensing or heating applications on the other hand work better when using a yarn with a lower conductivity. Conductive yarns are fabricated using either metallic wires or metalized textile yarns. Yarns can consist of a single fiber (monofilament) or can consist of various thinner fibers that are twisted together to form a composite fiber (multifilament). The conductivity of these yarns ranges from about 0.5 Ω/m to several kΩ/m, depending on the amount of metal used [88].

1.11 Need of binder free electrode

Wearable and fiber based devices have aroused a great interest in recent years because of their potential applications in stretchable energy and sensing applications [89, 90]. These substrates are easy-to-fabricate, mass-production and easy-to-use when compared to the conventional electrodes in practice such as FTO, ITO, Cu, stainless steel, Ni, Pt and metallic fillers. These metal and metallic fiber electrodes are limited by their self-oxidation and internal resistivity that easily influences the electrochemical activity. Usage of such electrode structures in electrochemical sensing enables the elimination of the use of insulating binders and conducting additives, which can greatly reduce contact resistance and the total mass of the electrode. Though binder is a necessary additive in traditional slurry-casting method, it can decrease the electrical conductivity, preventing the access of ions to the surface of active materials due to their insulating and electro-chemically inactive properties. This "dead surface" can block the contact with the electrolyte to actively participate in the electrochemical sensor. Hence, binder-free electrodes with the integration of unique merits of each component can provide larger electrochemically active surface area, faster electron transport and superior ion diffusion for high performance [91, 92].

1.12 Conductive carbon yarn

Carbon yarn, an outstanding class of carbon materials, has been widely applied in the field of electrochemistry and composite materials due to its intrinsic carrier mobility, electrical conductivity, environmental stability, superior mechanical properties, low weight, high temperature tolerance and low thermal expansion as well as potential for production at low cost [93-95]. In the yarn, the carbon atoms are bonded together in crystals that are more or less aligned parallel to the long axis of the fiber as the crystal alignment gives the fiber high strength-to-volume ratio [90]. These promising materials have also proved their potential applications in the fields including sensors, energy devices and flexible electronics [89, 92, 96].

With the boosting of nanomaterials and preparation technologies, different kinds of CF materials including CF fabric/textile/papers/webs, carbon nanofibers and carbon nanotubes (CNTs) fibers with diverse forms, compositions and microstructures have been developed [97-99]. Novel CF materials such as CNT fibers and graphene fibers can contain pure carbon atoms with carbon content as high as nearly 100% , which have demonstrated great potential in high-strength fibers, flexible conductors/electrodes, electrocatalysis, biosensing, and so on [100-102]. Fabrics based on conductive fibers represent an excellent class of substrates for developing wearable sensors because they would be in constant contact with the skin [103].

Therefore, integrating the surface of carbon fibers with the metal oxide based nanomaterials such as Fe_2O_3, SnO_2, TiO_2, ZnO, MnO_2, NiO, Carbon materials and conducting polymers can further enhance their electrochemical performances. Carbon cloth is usually used as a current collecting substrate to support metal oxides or conductive polymers because its network structure can provide rich active sites for electrochemical processes [104, 105]. Generally, the nanostructured metal oxide semiconductors possess high surface area, good biocompatibility, catalytic activity and chemical stability.

A choice of required materials is an important consideration for the development of wearable devices and the possibility to confer characteristic properties into the flexible and stretchable devices. The development of soft, flexible, semi-conductive or conductive material is essential for smart and wearable devices because of their unique chemical, mechanical and electronic, properties. Most widely used materials are metals and metal oxide NPs, nanowires (NWs), conductive polymers (CPs), carbon nanomaterials (CNMs) such as carbon particles, carbon fiber and CNTs and graphene, which have been studied.

1.13 Nanomaterials

"Nanotechnology is the understanding, control and manipulation of matter at dimensions of roughly 1 to 100 nanometers, where unique phenomena enable novel applications"

Nanoparticles size ranges between atoms and molecules and bulk. Therefore, a nanoparticle is defined as a particle with at least one dimension in the size range of

1-100 nm. By changing the size and shape of the nanomaterials, the properties like chemical, mechanical, physical, electronic, mechanical and magnetic varies from their bulk counterparts. Two major effects are responsible for shape and size dependent properties of nanostructures via increase in surface to volume ratio of nanostructures and quantum size effects, which influence their electronic structure. Based on the number of dimensions which are reduced to nanometer size range, nanomaterials are classified as zero-dimensional (quantum dots), one-dimensional (nanorods, nanowires, and nanotubules) and two-dimensional (graphene, quantum well, nanosheet) [106, 107].

Within nanomaterials, metal and semiconductor nanoparticles (NPs) are certainly the most studied and applied in electrochemical analysis. Such materials could be used to construct novel and improved sensing devices like electrochemical sensors and biosensors.

In the last decade nanostructured materials have experienced a rapid development due to their potential applications in a wide variety of technologies such as electronics, catalysis, ceramics, magnetic data storage, structural components, optoelectronic devices, display devices, biomaterials and gas/bio sensor [108, 109]. Such materials have s hown peculiar and fascinating physical, chemical and molecular properties along with applications performance superior to those of their bulk counterparts [109]. For electrochemical detection, nanomaterials play a very important role since they influence all aspects for electrochemical detection [110]. The immobilization of biological probes such as antibodies and DNA on to the sensor surface (conducing electrodes) requires highly specific binding chemistries, which may not be readily available on a native sensor surface. Nanomaterials can be used to provide the required functional sites for binding the probes to the sensor surface. The use of nanomaterials also significantly increases the surface-to-volume function at the sensor surface thereby leading to a high efficiency of antibody immobilization. For applications requiring high sensitivity and low detection limits, signal amplification is a key requirement and nanomaterials play an important role in amplifying the electrochemical response through improved electron transport at the sensor interface. Depending on the application and sensing technique, the dielectric properties and electrical conduction of the nanomaterial's can be tuned to amplify the response of the electrochemical signal [111].

1.13.1 Nanocomposites

The hybrid nanocomposites are a fast growing area of research in advanced functional materials science. Significant efforts have been focused on the ability to obtain nanostructures of desired shape, size, and properties using innovative synthetic approaches for various applications [112]. The properties of nanocomposite materials depend not only on the properties of their individual constituents, but also on their morphology and interfacial characteristics [113, 114]. The surface modification and functionalization of nanoparticles, covalent attachment, self-assembly and ease of organization on the surfaces provides a means to generate nanocomposite materials with tunable surface properties [115]. There is also a possibility of the realization of new properties that are unknown in the constituent materials. Efforts are continuing towards the preparation of new nanocomposite materials to obtain novel properties [116, 117].

1.13.2 Synthesis of nanomaterials

The properties of the particles generally depend on their size, shape, distribution and stabilizing agents, which are controlled by the preparatory conditions. This really allows us to think in both the "bottom up" (chemical method) or the "top down" (physical method) approaches (Fig. 1.9) to synthesize nanomaterials, i.e. either to assemble atoms together or to disassemble (break, or dissociate) bulk solids into finer pieces until they are constituted of only a few atoms [118, 119].

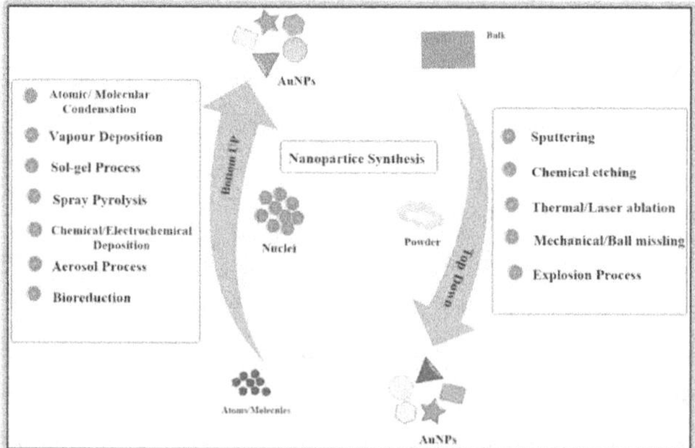

Fig. 1.9 Schematic illustrations of the preparative methods of nanoparticles

1.13.3 Hydrothermal method

Hydrothermal is the most important method to synthesis metal oxide and its composites, which is regarded as simple, safe and environmentally friendly. Other than that, hydrothermal method is believed to be used for producing smaller particles up to the nanoscale. Basically, hydrothermal reaction is carried out in stainless steel autoclave with Teflon liners under controlled temperature and pressure. This autoclave reaction will undergo a heating process via furnace heating or oven. The reaction occurs in aqueous solutions where water acts as a solvent. The temperatures can be elevated above the boiling point of water, reaching the pressure of vapor saturation. An internal pressure produced in this reaction is largely relative to the amount of solution added to the autoclave. According to earlier reports, with the help of reducing agents, various nanostructures were prepared successfully by hydrothermal method [120, 121].

1.13.4 Dip coating method

Dip coating is with no doubt the easiest and fast method to prepare the thin films from chemical solutions with the highest degree of control and also used for small scale production. In specific high technology cases, it is used to deposit coatings on large surfaces.

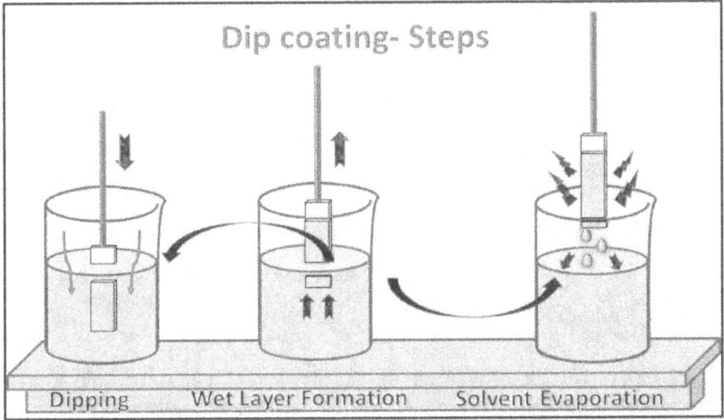

Fig. 1.10 Schematic illustration of dip coating method

The principle is as simple as dipping the substrate into the initial solution before withdrawing it at a constant speed. During this process, the solution naturally and homogeneously spreads out on the surface of the substrate by the combined effects of viscous drag and capillary rise. Evaporation then takes over and leads to solidification of the final coating. A fine tuning of the withdrawal speed and of the evaporation conditions (temperature and relative vapor pressure) is necessary to perfectly control the film characteristics (thickness and inner structure). The Schematic illustration of dip coating method is shown in Fig. 1.10. Amongst all available techniques used for such a purpose, the dip coating provides the unique and simple synthesis strategies [122, 123].

With these motivations, we have prepared metal oxide and carbon based electrodes as binder free immunoelectrodes for synergetic electrochemical cortisol sensing. The prepared materials were characterized using following analytical techniques.

1.14 Enzyme immobilization

Immobilization of enzymes is not a new concept but one that has been around for over 100 years. However, wide applications for immobilized enzymes came only in the past four decades in the form of synthesis of various complex drug intermediates; chemical synthesis under mild conditions without production of toxic by-products; remediation of polluted water, air and soil by removal of recalcitrant pollutant in an effective way; disease diagnosis; and correction of various genetic diseases due to the absence of metabolic enzymes, etc.

There are numerous methods for enzyme immobilization onto different materials that have been developed. Enzyme immobilization involves inclusion of enzymes into various matrices or binding onto their surfaces. Several modifications (e.g., pre-fabrication of matrices, enzyme cross-linking without addition of matrix) have been made and are still continuously evolving to update the protocols of immobilization so that immobilized enzymes become compatible for various emerging applications.

The properties of immobilized enzymes are determined by the type of enzyme and matrix used for the immobilization. Evolution of any new immobilization protocols focus primarily on: percentage enzyme recovery, operational stability, selectivity and reduction in inhibition by products or any other component present in the media. It involves intensive optimization of immobilization solutions to control the interaction between the matrix and the enzyme and proper orientation of the enzyme to maintain its catalytic properties [124].

1.14.1 Methods of enzyme immobilization

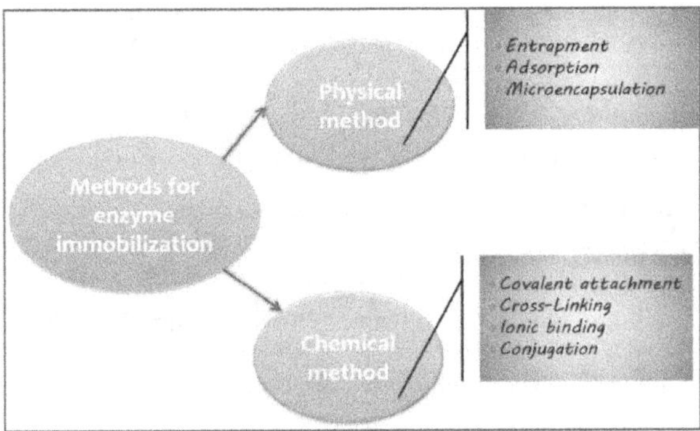

Fig. 1.11 Overview on the techniques being used for enzyme immobilization

Enzyme immobilization on the different matrices used to carry out via physical forces including van der Waals forces, hydrophobic interactions and hydrogen bonding (Fig. 1.11). The process is reversible in nature by controlling physico-chemical parameters. The other method involves chemical bonding like covalent or ionic bonds between the enzymes and matrices which is irreversible. Chemical interactions between antibodies and nanoparticle surface are achieved in the number of ways like (i) chemisorptions via thiol derivatives; (ii) through the use of bi-functional linkers) and through the use of adapter molecules like streptavidin and biotin.

1.14.2 Covalent binding

The enzyme is attached to the matrix by means of covalent bonds (diazotization, amino bond, Schiff's base formation, peptide bond and alkylation reactions). Enzyme molecules are attached either directly to the reactive groups (e.g., hydroxyl, amide, amino and carboxyl groups) present on the matrix or by a spacer arm, which is artificially attached to the matrix through various chemical reactions. Matrices commonly used are either natural (e.g., glass, Sephadex, Agarose and Sepharose) or synthetic (e.g., acrylamide, methacrylic acid and styrene). The selection of a particular matrix depends on its cost, availability, binding capacity, hydrophilicity, structural rigidity and durability during various applications. This method of immobilization involves non-essential amino acids (other than active site groups) leading to minimal conformational changes. It helps to promote the higher resistance of immobilized enzymes towards extreme physical and chemical conditions (e.g., temperature, denaturants and organic solvents). However, this method of immobilization leads to greater strain on the enzyme and sometimes leads to drastic changes in conformational and catalytic properties of the enzyme, due to harsh immobilization conditions and concurrence of similar amino-groups at the active site being involved during interaction of enzyme with the matrix [124].

1.14.3 Immobilization of cortisol monoclonal antibody using EDC/NHS chemistry

EDC (1-Ethyl-3-(3-dimethylaminopropyl)-carbodiimide) is a zero-length crosslinking agent used to couple carboxyl or phosphate groups to primary amines. This crosslinker has been used in diverse applications such as forming amide bonds in peptide synthesis, attaching heptanes to carrier proteins to form immunogens, labeling nucleic acids through 5' phosphate groups and creating amine-reactive NHS-esters of biomolecules.

One of the main advantages of EDC coupling is water soluble which allows direct bio-conjugation without prior organic solvent dissolution. On top of that, the excess of reagents and by-products can be easily removed by dialysis or gel-filtration. However, the coupling reaction has to be carried out fast, as the reactive ester that is formed can be rapidly hydrolyzed in aqueous solutions. To increase the stability of this active ester, N-hydroxysuccinimide (NHS) can be used. The addition of NHS stabilizes the amine-reactive intermediate by converting it to an amine-reactive NHS ester, thus increasing the efficiency of EDC-mediated coupling reactions. Key parameters that should be controlled when using EDC are the pH (as the hydrolysis is largely dependent on it) the amount of EDC so that nanoparticles do not aggregate due to loss of electrostatic repulsive forces among nanoparticles and the ratio of EDC/NHS [125, 126].

Adding NHS is just introducing an intermediate that is unstable, serves no practical purpose and reduces the yield if you are just crosslinking carboxyl groups to amino groups. Excess reagent and crosslinking by products can be easily removed by washing with water. Once EDC is water soluble, the crosslinking can be done under physiological conditions without adding any organic solvent.

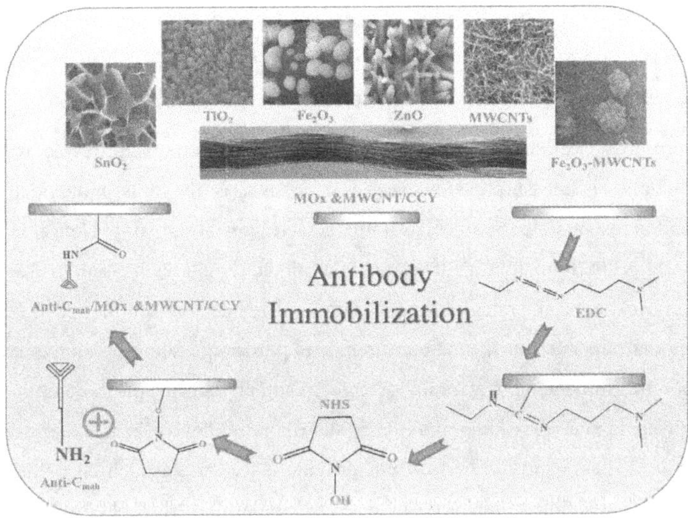

Fig. 1.12 Schematic illustration of immobilization of antibody on prepared electrodes

Using this protocol, almost all kinds of molecules (i.e. enzymes, antibodies, peptides, DNA, fluorophores, etc) can be attached to the nanoparticle surface without prior modification. Upon exposure of EDC/NHS to the carboxyl groups reactive NHS esters are formed. When a primary amine group in an antibody (or another protein) comes in contact with the ester, a covalent bond is formed. The successive immobilization steps of the present work are displayed in Fig. 1.12 [124, 127].

If the aim is to use nanostructured materials in immunosensor as biomarker detection, then, it is necessary to rightly choose the targeting component such as a monoclonal antibody, and the strategy to attach it on the surface of the particle. The electrodes conjugated by antibody or other functionalized groups have also been used as effective agents for POC applications.

1.15 Motivation of the work

Cortisol, a steroid hormone, is a biomarker for numerous diseases and plays an important role in the regulation of various physiological processes such as blood pressure, glucose levels, and carbohydrate metabolism, within the physiological limit. Since cortisol secretion is dependent on environmental and behavioral triggers, measurement of cortisol at POC has become imperative to understand behavioral patterns. Furthermore, normal levels of cortisol secretion follow a circadian rhythm with cortisol levels highest during daybreak and progressively lower as the day progresses.

Currently, in clinical practice, total cortisol, which is the sum of free and protein bound fractions, is measured. However, free cortisol is the only biologically active fraction and is responsible for all cortisol related activities in the body. Hence, in order to diagnose and properly treat cortisol-related conditions, regular estimation of free cortisol is required. Most current strategies for estimation of free cortisol are limited to laboratory techniques that are laborious, time-consuming, require large sample volume, expensive and cannot be implemented at point of care. Another significant shortcoming of the current set-up is that they only provide a snapshot of the cortisol levels of samples submitted in a diagnostic lab and do not provide a true representation of the cortisol variations that a specimen undergoes in an environment that triggers cortisol generation or suppression. Hence, real-time and continuous monitoring of cortisol levels is required to obtain valuable information that could assist doctors in better diagnosis and treatment of cortisol related conditions. Detection of 24-hour cortisol levels is currently a cumbersome process, which either involves admitting the patient for the time of study or where the patient samples blood/saliva into vials at specified time intervals during the 24-hour time period and ships it to a diagnostic laboratory. The typical turnaround time is 8 to 10 days and is still not a true representation of cortisol levels in stressful environments.

The application of POC requires wearable biosensors, which would open up a revolutionary opportunity to monitor even in remote areas which is a key for the development of modern healthcare. Wearable health monitoring technologies and devices are of great and continuous interest in clinical healthcare due to their ability to monitor physiological signals and to help maintain an optimal health status as well as assess the physical fitness of outpatients.

The researchers have made numerous efforts in order to address these inevitabilities in all areas including materials development, synthetic and immobilization strategies, prolonged time of processing and lack in accuracy. In spite of all these progresses made still there is room to develop new ideas and implementable strategies to tackle the issues.

In this regard, the development of sweat based cortisol sensor got significant attention in present scenario. The designing of efficient sensor electrodes is the prime factor in which new functional materials on flexible electrode platform employed in smart textiles.

With this motivation, we have made a new attempt to integrate the metal oxides and carbon material on conductive carbon yarn using simple synthesis routes. The analysis part gave us a brief insight on material properties to meet out the sensor perspectives.

1.16 Objectives of the present work

The specific objectives of the present research includes,

- Synthesis and integration of various morphological metal oxides (Fe_2O_3, ZnO, TiO_2, SnO_2) on carbon fibers using chemical hydrothermal route

- Functionalization and incorporation of MWCNTs and hybrids onto the CCY through simple dip coating method.

- Evaluation of physico-chemical properties of the prepared nanomaterials using various analytical techniques and understanding their influences in immunosensing performance.

- Investigation of redox behavior of prepared metal oxides, their surface features and mechanical properties influencing the detection of biomarker.

- Analyzing the immobilization kinetics of monoclonal cortisol antibodies on the developed fiber based electrodes.

- Explore and identify the better electrochemical efficacy of the prepared immunoelectrodes towards the detection of cortisol.

- Measurement of cortisol levels in human sweat and validation of the sensor results with commercial chemiluminescence immunoassay (CLIA) method for real time applications.

References

1. A. Qureshi, Y. Gurbuz, J. H. Niazi, Biosensors for cardiac biomarkers detection: A review, *Sens. Actuator B-Chem,* **171–172** (2012) 62–76.

2. J. L. Martin-Ventura, L. M. Blanco-Colio, J. Tunon, B. Munoz-Garcia, J. Madrigal Matute, J. A. Moreno, M. Vega de Ceniga, J. Egido, Biomarkers in cardiovascular medicine, *Rev Esp Cardiol.,* **62** (2009) 677–688.

3. M. C. N. Bairey, J. Dwyer, C. K. Nordstrom, K. G. Walton, J. W. Salerno, R. H. Schneider, Psychosocial stress and cardiovascular disease: pathophysiological links, *Behav Med.,* **27** (2002) 141–147

4. S. Anastasova, B. Crewther, P. Bembnowicz, V. Curto, H. MD Ip, B. Rosa, G. Z. A. Yang, Wearable multisensing patch for continuous sweat monitoring, *Biosens. Bioelectron.,* **93** (2017) 139–145.

5. T. Kamei, T. Tsuda, S. Kitagawa, K. Naitoh, K. Nakashima, T. Ohhashi, Physical stimuli and emotional stress-induced sweat secretions in the human palm and forehead, *Anal. Chim. Acta,* **365** (1998) 319–326.

6. A. P. F. Turner, Biosensors: Sense and sensibility, *Chem. Soc. Rev.,* **42** (2013) 3184–3196.

7. D. Son, J. Lee, S. Qiao, R. Ghaffari, J. Kim, J. E. Lee, C. Song, S. J. Kim, D. J. Lee, S. W. Jun, S. Yang, M. Park, J. Shin, K. Do, M. Lee, K. Kang, C. S. Hwang, N. Lu, T. Hyeon, D. H. Kim, Multifunctional wearable devices for diagnosis and therapy of movement disorders, *Nat. Nanotechnol.,* **9** (2014) 397–404.

8. E. R. de Kloet, J. M. Holsboer Florian, Stress and the brain: from adaptation to disease, *Nat Rev Neurosci.,* **6** (2005) 463-475.

9. A. Levine, O. Zagoory-Sharon, R. Feldman, J. G. Lewis, A. Weller, Measuring cortisol in human psychobiological studies, *Physiol. Behav.,* **90** (2007) 43–53.

10. S. K. Arya, G. Chornokur, M. Venugopal, S. Bhansali, Dithiobis(succinimidyl propionate) modified gold microarray electrode based electrochemical immunosensor for ultrasensitive detection of cortisol, *Biosens. Bioelectron,* **25** *(2010)* 2296–2301.

11. M. D. Corbalan-Tutau, J. A. Madrid, F. Nicolas, M. Garaulet, Daily profile in two circadian markers "melatonin and cortisol" and associations with metabolic syndrome components, *Physiol Behav.*, **123** (2014) 231-235 .

12. F. Holsboer and M. Ising, Stress hormone regulation: biological role and translation into therapy, *Annu. Rev. Clin. Psychol.*, **61** (2010) 81-109.

13. B. S. McEwen, Cortisol, Cushing's syndrome, and a shrinking brain-New evidence for reversibility, *J. Clin. Endocrinol. Metab.*, **87** (2002) 1947-1948.

14. O. Edwards, J. M. Galley, R. J. Courtenay-Evans, J. Hunter, A. Tait, Changes in cortisol metabolism following rifampicin therapy, *Lancet.*, **2** (1974) 548-551.

15. S. J. Lupien, B. S. McEwen, M. R. Gunnar, C. Heim, Effects of stress throughout the lifespan on the brain, behaviour and cognition, *Nat. Rev. Neurosci.*, **10** (2009) 434 445.

16. F. Holsboer and M. Ising, Stress hormone regulation: biological role and translation into therapy, *Annu. Rev. Psychol.*, **61** (2010) 81–109.

17. M. Venugopal, S. K. Arya, G. Chornokur, S. Bhansali, A Real time and Continuous Assessment of Cortisol in ISF Using Electrochemical Impedance Spectroscopy, *Sens Actuators A – Phys,* **172** (2011) 154–160.

18. Z. Djuric, C. E. Bird, A. Furumoto-Dawson, G. H. Rauscher, M. T. Ruffin Iv, R. P. Stowe, K. L. Tucker, C. M. Masi, Biomarkers of psychological stress in health disparities research. *Open Biomark. J,* **1** (2008) 7–19.

19. S. Anastasova, B. Crewther, P. Bembnowicz, V. Curto, H. MD Ip, B. Rosa, G. Z. A. Yang, wearable multisensing patch for continuous sweat monitoring, *Biosens. Bioelectron.,* **93** (2017) 139–145.

20. H. Dobson and R. F. Smith, What is stress, and how does it affect reproduction?, *Anim. Reproduct. Sci.,* **60-61** (2000) 743–752.

21. R. D. Munje, S. Muthukumar, A. PanneerSelvam, S. Prasad, Flexible nanoporous tunable electrical double layer biosensors for sweat diagnostics, *Sci. Rep.,* 5 (2015) 14586.

22. J. Brossaud, D. Ducint, B. Gatta, M. Molimard, A. Tabarin, J. Corcuff, Urinary cortisol metabolites in corticotroph and adrenal tumours, *Endocr. Abstr* **50** (2012) PL1.

23. M. Venugopal, K. E. Feuvrel, D. Mongin, S. Bambot, M. Faupel, A. Panangadan, A. Talukder, R. Pidva, Clinical evaluation of a novel interstitial fluid sensor system for remote continuous alcohol monitoring, *Sensors J. IEEE,* **8** (2008) 71–80.

24. E. V. Mukerjee, S. D. Collins, R. V. Isseroff, R. L. Smith, Micro needle array for transdermal biological fluid extraction and in situ analysis, *Sensors Actuat. A: Phys.* **114** (2004) 267–275.

25. P. M. Wang, M. Cornwell, M. R. Prasunitz, Minimally invasive extraction of dermal interstitial fluid for glucose monitoring using microneedles, *Diabetes Technol. Ther.,* **7** (2005) 131–141.

26. A. Bennett and V. Hayssen, Hair as a biological indicator of drug use, drug abuse or chronic exposure to environmental toxicants, *Int J Toxicol.,* **25** (2006) 143-63.

27. L. Koren, O. Mokady, T. Karaskov, J. Klein, G. Koren, E. Geffen, A novel method using hair for determining hormonal levels in wildlife. *Animal Behaviour,* **63** (2002) 403-406.

28. B. Sauvé, G. Koren, G. Walsh, S. Tokmakejian, S. H. V. Uum, Measurement of cortisol in human hair as a biomarker of systemic exposure, *Clin Invest Med.,* **30** (2007) 83-91.

29. W. Gao, Q. Xie, J. Jina, T. Qiao, H. Wang, L. Chen, H. Deng, Z. Lua, HPLC-FLU detection of cortisol distribution in human hair, *Clin Biochem.,* **43** (2010) 677-682.

30. J. S. Raul, V. Cirimele, B. Ludes, P. Kintz, Detection of physiological concentrations of cortisol and cortisone in human hair, *Clin Biochem.,* **37** (2004) 1105-1111.

31. R. Gow, S. Thomson, M. Rieder, S. V. Uum, G. Koren An assessment of cortisol analysis in hair and its clinical applications, *Forensic Sci Int.,* **196** (2010) 32-37.

32. C. W. L. Roux, G. Chapman, W. Kong, W. Dhillo, J. Jones, J. A. Zadeh, Free cortisol index is better than serum total cortisol in determining hypothalamic-pituitary-adrenal status in patients undergoing surgery, *J. Clin. Endocrinol. Metab.,* **88** (2003) 2045-2048.

33. A. Levine, O. Z. Sharon, R. Feldman, J. G. Lewis, A. Weller, Measuring cortisol in human psychobiological studies, *Physiol. Behav.,* **90** (2007) 43–53.

34. M. D.V. Bruggen, A. C. Hackney, R. G. McMurra, K. S. Ondrak, The relationship between serum and salivary cortisol levels in response to different intensities of exercise, *Int J Sports Physiol. Perform.,* **6** (2011) 396–407.

35. T. Umeda, R. Hiramatsu, T. Iwaoka, T. Shimada, F. Miura, T. Sato, Use of saliva for monitoring unbound free cortisol levels in serum, *Clin. Chim. Acta,* **110** (1981) 245-253.

36. E. V. Caenegem, K. Wierckx, T. Fiers, H. Segers, E. Vandersypt, J. M. Kaufman, G. T. Sjoen, Salivary cortisol and testosterone: a comparison of salivary sample collection methods in healthy controls, *Endocr. Abstr,* **26** (2011) P355.

37. D. Price, G. Close, B. Fielding, Age of appearance of circadian rhythmin salivary cortisol values in infancy, *Arch. Dis. Child.,* **58** (1983) 454–456.

38. H. Raff, J. L. Raff, J. W. Findling, Late-night salivary cortisol as a screening test for Cushing's syndrome, *J. Clin. Endocrinol. Metab.,* **83** (1998) 2681-2686.

39. K. Løvås, T. Thorsen, E. Husebye, Saliva cortisol measurement: simple and reliable assessment of the glucocorticoid replacement therapy in Addison's disease. *J Endocrinol Invest.,* **29** (2006) 727-731.

40. A. Granger, A. Henry, L. Lilliencrantz, A. Smith, P. Srnis, W. V. Schepen, E. Injeti, Effects of physical stress and maturational changes on hypothalamic pituitary adrenal axis function through cortisol analysis (2012).

41. L. L. Carpenter, T. T. Shattuck, A. R. Tyrka, T. D. Geraciot, L. H. Price, Effect of childhood physical abuse on cortisol stress response, *Psychopharmacology,* **214** (2011) 367-375.

42. H. Prunty, K. Andrews, G. R. Kolanu, P. Quinlan, P. Wood, Sweat patch cortisol-a new screen for Cushing's syndrome, *Endocr. Abstr,* (2004) **P202**.

43. E. Russell, G. Koren, M. Reider, S. V. Uum, The detection of cortisol in human sweat: implications for measurement of cortisol in hair, *Endocr. Rev.,* **36** (2012) 30-34.

44. K. Mitsubayashi, M. Suzuki, E. Tamiya, I. Karube, Analysis of metabolites in sweat as a measure of physical condition, *Anal. Chim. Acta*, **289** (1994) 27–34.

45. M. F. Bergeron, Heat cramps: fluid and electrolyte challenges during tennis in the heat, *J. Sci. Med. Sport.*, **6** (2003) 19–27.

46. R. C. Stern, The diagnosis of cystic fibrosis, *N. Engl. J. Med.*, **336** (1997) 487–49.

47. Pilardeau, P. Pilardeau, J. Vaysse, M. Garnier, M. Joublin, L. Valeri, Secretion of eccrine sweat glands during exercise, *Br. J. Sports Med.*, **13** (1979) 118–121.

48. R. P. Heaney, Calcium in the prevention and treatment of osteoporosis, *J. Int. Med.*, **231** (1992) 169–180.

49. R. C. Klesge, K. D. Ward, M. L. Shelton, W. B. Applegate, E. D. Cantler, G. M. Palmieri, K. Harmon, J. Davis, Changes in bone mineral content in male athletes mechanisms of action and intervention effects, *J. Am. Med. Assoc.*, **276** (1996) 226–230.

50. M. Gamella, S. Campuzano, J. Manso, G. G. deRivera, F. L. Colino, A. J. Reviejo, J. M. Pingarrón, A novel non-invasive electrochemical biosensing device for in situ determination of the alcohol content in blood by monitoring ethanol in sweat, *Anal. Chim. Acta*, **806** (2014) 1–7.

51. M. Burns and C. Baselt, Monitoring drug use with a sweat patch: an experiment with cocaine, *J. Anal. Toxicol.*, **19** (1995) 41–48.

52. A. Kaushik, A. Vasudev, S. K. Arya, S. K. Pasha, S. Bhansali, Recent advances in cortisol sensing technologies for point-of-care application, *Biosens. Bioelectron.*, **53** (2014) 499-512.

53. U. Turpeinen, H. Markkanen, M. Välimäki, U. H. Stenman, Determination of urinary free cortisol by HPLC, *Clin. Chem.*, **43** (1997) 1386-1391.

54. P. M. Kabra, L. L. Tsai, L. J. Marton, Improved liquid-chromatographic method for determination of serum cortisol, *Clin Chem.*, **25** (1979) 1293–1296.

55. G. E. Abraham, J. E. Buster, R.C. Teller, Radioimmunoassay of plasma cortisol, *Anal. Lett.*, **5** (1972) 757-765.

56. H. J. Ruder, R. L. Guy, M. B. Lipsett, A radioimmunoassay for cortisol in plasma and urine, *J. Clin. Endocrinol. Metab.,* **35** (1972) 219-224.

57. M. Kao, S. Voina, A. Nichols, R. Horton, Parallel radioimmunoassay for plasma cortisol and 11-deoxycortisol, *Clin.Chem.,* **21** (1975) 1644-1647.

58. R. J. Dash, B. G. England, A. R. Midgley, G. D. Niswender, A specific, non-chromatographic radioimmunoassay for human plasma cortisol, *Steroids,* **26** (1975) 647-661.

59. Y. Kobayashi, K. Amitani, F. Watanabe, K. Miyai, Fluorescence polarization immunoassay for cortisol, *Clin. Chim. Acta,* **92** (1979) 241-247.

60. D. Appel, R. D. Schmid, C. A. Dragan, M. Bureik, V. B. Urlacher, A fluorimetric assay for cortisol, *Anal. Bioanal. Chem.,* **383** (2005) 182-186.

61. C. Carrozza, S. M. Corsello, R. M. Paragliola, F. Ingraudo, S. Palumbo, P. Locantore, A. Sferrazza, A. Pontecorvi , C. Zuppi, Clinical accuracy of midnight salivary cortisol measured by automated electrochemiluminescence immunoassay method in Cushing's syndrome, *Ann Clin Biochem.,* **47** (2010) 228-232.

62. M. Yaneva, G. Kirilov, S. Zacharieva, Midnight salivary cortisol, measured by highly sensitive electrochemiluminescence immunoassay, for the diagnosis of Cushing's syndrome, *Eur J Med Res.,* **4** (2009) 59-64.

63. Z. E. Belaya, A. V. Iljin, G. A. Melnichenko, L. Y. Rozhinskaya, N. V. Dragunova, L. K. Dzeranova, S. A. Butrova, E. A. Troshina, I. I. Dedov, Diagnostic performance of late-night salivary cortisol measured by automated electrochemiluminescence immunoassay in obese and overweight patients referred to exclude Cushing's syndrome, *Endocrine,* **41** (2012) 494-500.

64. G. Lippi, F. D. Vita, G. L. Salvagno, M. Gelati, M. Montagnana, G. C. Guidi, Measurement of morning saliva cortisol in athletes, *Clin Biochem.,* **42** (2009) 904-906.

65. P. Pervanidou, G. Kolaitis, S. Charitaki, C. Lazaropoulou, I. Papassotiriou, P. Hindmarsh, C. Bakoula, J. Tsiantis, G. P. Chrousos, The natural history of neuroendocrine changes in pediatric posttraumatic stress disorder (PTSD) after motor vehicle accidents: Progressive divergence of noradrenaline and cortisol concentrations over time, *Biol Psychiatry.,* **62** (2007) 1095-1102.

66. A. L. McRae, M. E. Saladin, K. T. Brady, H. Upadhyaya, S. E. Back, M. A. Timmerman, Stress reactivity: biological and subjective responses to the cold pressor and Trier Social stressors, *Hum Psychopharmacol.*, **21** (2006) 377-385.

67. J. Lewis and P. Elder, An enzyme-linked immunosorbent assay (ELISA) for plasma cortisol, *Biochem Mol Biol.*, **22** (1985) 673-676.

68. M. Shimada, K. Takahashi, T. Ohkawa, M. Segawa, M. Higurashi, Determination of salivary cortisol by ELISA and its application to the assessment of the circadian rhythm in children, *Horm Res.*, **44** (1995) 213-217.

69. B. C. Small and K.B. Davis, Validation of a time-resolved fluoroimmunoassay for measuring plasma cortisol in channel catfish ictalurus punctatus, *J. World Aquacult Soc.*, **33** (2007) 184-187.

70. M. A. Cooper, Label-free screening of bio-molecular interactions, *Anal Bioanal Chem.*, **377** (2003) 834-842.

71. D. R. Shankaran, K.V. Gobi, N. Miura, Recent advancements in surface plasmon resonance immunosensors for detection of small molecules of biomedical, food and environmental interest, *Sens. Actuator B-Chem.*, **121** (2007) 158-177.

72. J. S. Mitchell, T.E. Lowe, J.R. Ingram, Rapid ultrasensitive measurement of salivary cortisol using nano-linker chemistry coupled with surface Plasmon resonance detection, *Analyst,* **134** (2008) 380-386.

73. R. C. Stevens, S. D. Soelberg, S. Near, C. E. FurlongDetection of cortisol in saliva with a flow-filtered, portable surface plasmon resonance biosensor system, *Anal. Chem.*, **80** (2008) 6747-6751.

74. M. Z. Atashbar, B. Bejcek, A. Vijh, S. Singamaneni, QCM biosensor with ultra thin polymer film, *Sens. Actuator B-Chem.*, **107** (2005) 945-951.

75. F. Ricci, G. Adornetto, G. Palleschi, A review of experimental aspects of electrochemical immunosensors, *Electrochim. Acta,* **84** (2012) 74–83.

76. Y. Wan, Y. Su, X. Zhu, G. Liu, C. Fan, Development of electrochemical immunosensors towards point of care diagnostics, *Biosens. Bioelectron.*, **47** (2013) 1–11.

77. Y. F. Ricci, G. Adornetto, G. Palleschi, A review of experimental aspects of electrochemical immunosensors, *Electrochim. Acta,* **84** (2012) 74–83.

78. Z. I. H. Cho, J. Lee, J. Kim, M. S. Kan, J. K. Paik, S. Ku, H. M. Cho, J. Irudayaraj, D. H. Kim, Current Technologies of Electrochemical Immunosensors: Perspective on Signal Amplification, *Sensors,* **18** (2018) 207 (1-18)

79. D. Purvis, O. Leonardova, D. Farmakovsky, V. Cherkasov, An ultrasensitive and stable potentiometric immunosensor, *Biosens. Bioelectron.,* **18** (2003) 1385-1390.

80. Y. Ni, Y. Wang and S. Kokot, Simultaneous determination of three fluoroquinolones by linear sweep stripping voltammetry with the aid of chemometrics, *Talanta,* **69** (2006) 216-225.

81. R. S. Nicholson, Theory and application of cyclic voltammetry for measurement of electrode reaction kinetics, *Anal. Chem.,* **37** (1965) 1351- 1355.

82. R. Gatti, G. Antonelli, M. Prearo, P. Spinella, E. Cappellin, E. F. De Palo, Cortisol assay sand diagnostic laboratory procedures in human biological fluids, *Clin. Biochem.,* **42** (2009) 1205–1217.

83. D. L. Delahanty, A. J. Raimonde, E. Spoonster, Initial post traumatic urinary cortisol levels predict subsequent PTSD symptoms in motor vehicle accident victims, *Biol. Psychiatry,* **48** (2000) 940–947.

84. R. Yehuda, S. L. Halligan, L. M. Bierer, Cortisol levels in adult offspring of Holocaust survivors: relation to PTSD symptom severity in the parent and child. *Psychoneuroendocrinology,* **27** (2002) 171–180.

85. W. Gao, S. Emaminejad, H. Y. Y. Nyein, S. Challa, K. Chen, A. Peck, H. M. Fahad, H. Ota, H. Shiraki, D. Kiriya, D. H. Lien, G. A. Brooks, R. W. Davis, A. Javey, Fully integrated wearable sensor arrays for multiplexed in situ perspiration analysis, *Nature,* **529** (2016) 209-514.

86. O. Parlak, S. T. Keene, A. Marais, V. F. Curto, A. Salleo, Molecularly selective nanoporous membrane-based wearable organic electrochemical device for noninvasive cortisol sensing, *Sci. Adv.,* **4** (2018) 1-10.

87. K. Cherenack and L. V. Pieterson, Smart textiles: Challenges and opportunities, *J. Appl. Phys.*, **112** (2012) 091301(1-14).

88. C. Randell, S. Baurley, M. Chalmers, and H. Muller, Textile tools for wearable computing, *Proceedings of the International Forum on Applied Wearable Computing, 1395 (IFAWC 2004)*, 2004.

89. D. P. Hansora, N.G. Shimpi, S. Mishraa, Performance of hybrid nanostructured conductive cotton materials as wearable devices: an overview of materials, fabrication, properties and applications, *RSC Adv.*, **5** (2015) 107716–107770.

90. S. Chand, Carbon fibers for composites, *J. Mater. Sci.*, **35** (2000) 1303–1313.

91. G. Zhou, F. Li, H.M. Cheng, Progress in flexible lithium batteries and future prospects, *Energy Environ. Sci.*, **7** (2014) 1307–1338.

92. S. Madhu, P. Manickam, M. Pierre, S. Bhansali, P. Nagamony, V. Chinnuswamy, Nanostructured SnO_2 integrated conductive fabrics as binder-free electrode for neurotransmitter detection, *Sens. Actuator A-Phys*, **269** (2018) 401–411.

93. Y. Zhang, Z. Hu, Y. Liang, Y. Yang, N. An, Z. Li, H. Wu, Growth of 3D SnO_2 nanosheets on carbon cloth as a binder-free electrode for supercapacitors, *J. Mater. Chem. A*, **3** (2015) 15057–15067.

94. Y. Liu, X. Fang, M. Ge, J. Rong, C. Shen, A. Zhang, H. A. Enaya, C. Zhou, SnO_2 coated carbon cloth with surface modification as Na-ion battery anode, *Nano Energy*, **16** (2015) 399–407.

95. J. Bai, P. Qi, X. Ding, H. Zhang, Graphene composite coated carbon fiber: electrochemical synthesis and application in electrochemical sensing, *RSC Adv.*, **6** (2016) 11250–11255.

96. B. S. Shim, W. Chen, C. Doty, C. Xu, N. Kotov, A. Smart electronic yarns and wearable fabrics for human biomonitoring made by carbon nanotube coating with polyelectrolytes. *Nano Lett.*, **8** (2008) 4151–4157.

97. Q. Zhang, J. P. Rong, D. S. Ma and B. Q. Wei, The governing self-discharge processes in activated carbon fabric-based supercapacitors with different organic electrolyte, *Energy Environ. Sci.*, **4** (2011) 2152-2159.

98. X. H. Lu, T. Zhai, X. H. Zhang, Y. Q. Shen, L. Y. Yuan, B. Hu, L. Gong, J. Chen, Y. H. Gao, J. Zhou, Y. X. Tong and Z. L. Wang, WO_3–x@Au@MnO_2 Core–Shell nanowires on carbon fabric for high-performance flexible supercapacitors, *Adv. Mater.*, **24** (2012) 938-944.

99. M. Endo, Y. A. Kim, T. Hayashi, K. Nishimura, T. Matusita, K. Miyashita and M. S. Dresselhaus, Vapor-grown carbon fibers (VGCFs): Basic properties and their battery applications, *Carbon,* **39** (2001) 1287-1297.

100. W. B. Lu, M. Zu, J. H. Byun, B. S. Kim and T. W. Chou, State of the art of carbon nanotube fibers: opportunities and challenges, *Adv. Mater.*, **24** (2012) 1805-1833.

101. J. Foroughi, G. M. Spinks, G. G. Wallace, J. Oh, M. E. Kozlov, S. Fang, T. Mirfakhrai, J.D. W. Madden, M. K. Shin, S. J. Kim and R. H. Baughman, Torsional carbon nanotube artificial muscles, *Science,* **334** (2011) 494-497.

102. G. X. Qu, J. L. Cheng, X. D. Li, D. M. Yuan, P. N. Chen, X. L. Chen, B. Wang, H. S. Peng, A Fiber Supercapacitor with High Energy Density Based on Hollow Graphene/Conducting Polymer Fiber Electrode, *Adv. Mater.*, **28** (2016) 3646-3652.

103. S. Pasche, S. Angeloni, R. Ischer, M. Liley, J. Luprano, G. Voirin, Wearable biosensors for monitoring wound healing, *Adv. Sci. Technol.,* **57** (2008) 80–87.

104. Y. Zhang, H. Zhongai, Y. Liang, Y. Yang, N. An, Z. Li, W. Hongying, Growth of 3D SnO_2 nanosheets on carbon cloth as a binder-free electrode for supercapacitors, *J. Mater. Chem. A,* **3** (2015) 15057–15067.

105. K. P. O. Mahesh, I. Shown, L. C. Chen, K. H. Chen, Y. Tai, Flexible sensor for dopamine detection fabricated by the direct growth of α-Fe_2O_3 nanoparticles on carbon cloth, *Appl. Surf. Sci.,* **427** (2018) 387–395.

106. M. M. Rahman- Nanomaterials, *Publisher: InTech* **(2011)** *ISBN 9789533079134356.*

107. R. W. Kelsall, I. W. Hamley, M. Geoghegan, Nanoscale science and technology, *John Wiley & Sons, Ltd,* **(2005),** *ISBN:9780470850862*

108. F. Caruso, Nanoengineering of Particle Surfaces, *Adv. Mater.,* **13** (2001) 11-22.

109. A. Nabok, Organic and inorganic nanostructures, *Publisher: Artech House Publishers,* **(2005)** *ISBN: 978-1580538190*

110. J. Wang, Nanomaterial-based electrochemical biosensors, *Analyst,* **130** (2005) 421-426.

111. J. Wang, Nanomaterial-based amplified transduction of biomolecular interactions, *Small,* **1** (2005) 1036-1043.

112. G. Carotenuto, L. Nicolais, B. Martorana, P. Perlo, Metal-Polymer Nanocomposite Synthesis: Novel ex situ and in situ Approaches, in Metal–Polymer Nanocomposites, *Publisher: John Wiley & Sons,* Inc (2005), ISBN: 978-0471695431.

113. P. G. Romero, M. Chojak, K. C. Gallegos, J. A. Asensio, P. J. Kulesza, N. C. Pastora, M. L. Cantú, Hybrid organic–inorganic nanocomposite materials for application in solid state electrochemical supercapacitors, *Electrochem. Commun.,* **5** (2003) 149-153.

114. J. Shi, Z. Hua, L.X Zhang, Nanocomposites from ordered mesoporous materials. *J. Mater. Chem.,* **14** (2004) 795-806.

115. P Manivel, S Kanagaraj, A Balamurugan, N Ponpandian, D Mangalaraj, C Viswanathan, Rheological behavior and electrical properties of polypyrrole/thermally reduced graphene oxide nanocomposite, *Colloids Surf. A,* **441** (2014) 614-622

116. C. Nastase, F.Nastase, A. Vaseashta, I. Stamatin,Nanocomposites based on functionalized nanotubes in polyaniline matrix by plasma polymerization, *Prog. Solid State Chem.,* **34** (2006) 181-189.

117. R. Sriramprabha, M. Divagar, N. Ponpandian, C. Viswanathan, Tin Oxide/Reduced graphene oxide nanocomposite-modified electrode for selective and sensitive detection of riboflavin, *J. Electrochem. Soc.,* **165** (2018) B498-B507.

118. A. Sengupta, C. K. Sarkar, Introduction to Nano-Basics to Nanoscience and Nanotechnology, *Springer publication* **(2015)** ISBN 978-3-662-47314-6.

119. A. Inmaculada, L. Lorente, M. Valcarcel, Analytical Nanoscience and technology, *Compr Anal Chem,* **66** (2014) 3-35.

120. D. A. Palmer, R. F. Prini, A. H. Harvey, Aqueous systems at elevated temperatures and pressures, *Publisher: Elsevier* **(2004)** *ISBN-978-0-12-544461-3.*

121. P. G. Jessop, W. Leitner, Chemical synthesis using supercritical fluids, *Publisher: Wiley VCH* **(2007)** ISBN: 978-3527296057.

122. J. Feng, H. Xia, F. Mao Alignment of Ag nanowires on glass sheet by dip coating techniques, *J. Alloys Compd.,* **735** (2018) 607-612.

123. M. E. Spotnitz, D. Ryan, H. A. Stone, Dip coating for the alignment of carbon nanotubes on curved surfaces, *J. Mater. Chem.,* **14** (2004) 1299-1302.

124. A. Dwevedi, Enzyme Immobilization: Advances in Industry, Agriculture, Medicine and the Environment, **Publisher: Springer** (2016) *ISBN 978-3-319-41418-8.*

125. 1. J. Conde, A. Ambrosone, V. Sanz, Y. Hernández, V. Marchesano, F. Tian, H. Child, C.C. Berry, M.R. Ibarra, P.V. Baptista, C. Tortiglione, J. M. Fuente, Design of Multifunctional Gold Nanoparticles for in vitro and in vivo Gene Silencing, *ACS Nano,* **6** (2012) 8316–8324.

126. V. Sanz, João Conde, Y. Hernández, P.V. Baptista, M.R. Ibarra and J. M. de la Fuente, Effect of PEG biofunctional spacers and TAT peptide on dsRNA loading on Gold Nanoparticles, *J Nanopart Res,* **14** (2012) 1-9.

127. J. Conde, P.V. Baptista, Y. Hernández, V. Sanz and J.M. de la Fuente, Modification of Plasmid DNA Topology by Histone-Mimetic Gold Nanoparticles, *Nanomedicine,* **7** (2012) 1657-1666.

Chapter II

Nanostructured SnO₂ Integrated Conductive Fibers as Binder-Free Electrodes for Cortisol Measurement

Highlights

> ➤ New attempt has been made to deposit SnO_2 nanostructures onto carbon yarns using simple hydrothermal method.

> ➤ SnO_2 integrated carbon fibers were directly used as binder-free electrodes for electrochemical detection of cortisol.

> ➤ SnO_2 coated carbon yarns were showed good adhesion property.

> ➤ Involvement of external redox mediator has been avoided, which would prolong the utility period of the sensor electrode.

> *Graphical illustration of immobilization and electrochemical immunosensing of cortisol on hydrothermally derived SnO₂/CCY with possible redox mechanism*

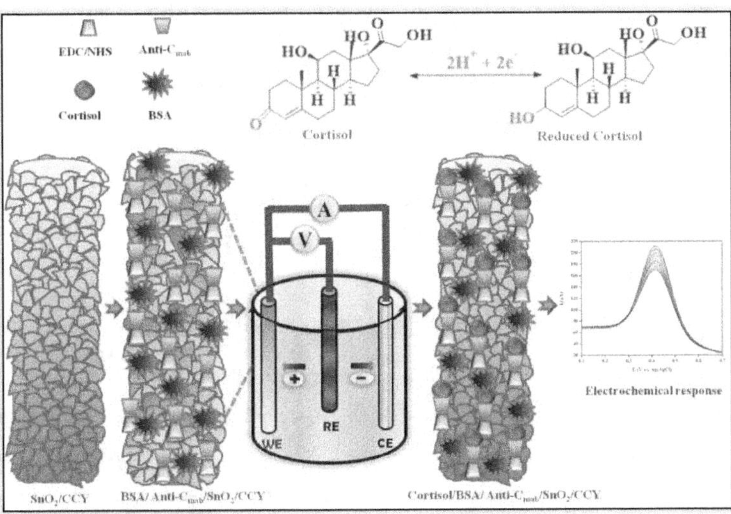

2.1 Introduction

Metal oxides are the source of functional materials that have tunable properties and significant technological applications [1]. Tin oxide (SnO_2) is an n-type semiconductor metal oxide with wide energy gap (E= 3.62 eV, at 300 K). SnO_2 has high chemical stability, high surface area to volume ratio and found have applications in wide varieties of research areas such as solar cells, energy storage devices, electrochemical sensors, biosensors, gas sensors and photocatalysis, etc., [2-4]. Physical and chemical properties of nanocrystalline SnO_2 are often differ from its bulk and amorphous counterparts. The crystal structure of the SnO_2 is shown in Fig. 2.1. The physico-chemical properties are greatly influenced by particle size, morphology, and crystal structure. Thus, the synthesis of SnO_2 nanostructures with desired morphology is of great technological and scientific interest owing to their superior physical and chemical properties [5, 6]. Recently, numbers of efforts have been devoted to formulate the nanostructures of SnO_2 with different morphologies for tuning their specific surface area, sensitivity and efficiency [7].

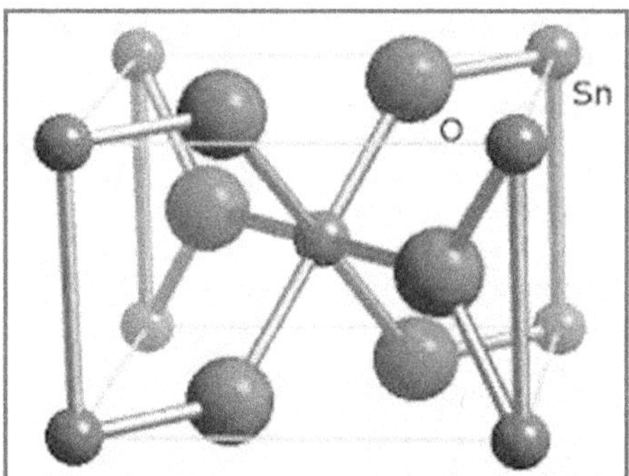

Fig. 2.1 The structure of nanocrystalline SnO_2

Various methods including sol-gel, co-precipitation, evaporation, sputtering, hydrothermal and ultrasonic spray pyrolysis [8-10] have been investigated to prepare the SnO_2 nanostructures with desired morphologies. Among many preparative methods, the hydrothermal method is widely used due to its simplicity, product purity and low cost. The major advantages of using this process is utilization of low to medium temperatures under controlled pressures compared to the other conventional synthesis processes which require medium to high temperature range. Indeed, the morphologies of the nanostructures can also be tuned by changing experimental parameters.

Integration of SnO_2 nanostructures with the electrode surface found to enhance the electrochemical characteristics of the electrodes. For example, Koichi Ui *et al.,* (2012) fabricated the binder-free SnO_2 anode material for LIB's by an electrophoretic deposition method and examined its morphological influence on its electrochemical characteristics. [13]. Zhang *et al.,* (2015) coated carbon cloth (CC) with SnO_2 nanoflakes and achieved a specific capacitance of 247 F g^{-1} [14]. Cheng *et al.,* (2011) coated polyaniline (PANI) nanowires on CC and attained a normalized specific capacitance of 673 F g^{-1}. The resulting SnO_2/CC and PANI/CC can directly be used as a binder-free (or redox-mediator free) electrode without any additives or external redox probes which limits the charge transfer and active ion diffusion of the electrode material [15]. Y. Liu *et al.,* (2015) have reported that the SnO_2 coated carbon cloth can be used as Na-ion battery anode for battery applications. The SnO_2 modified electrodes exhibited superior electrochemical properties, when compare than reported values [16].

SnO_2 nanotubular materials have been prepared using natural cellulose fibers as template for gas sensing applications. The gas sensor platform was fabricated using the SnO_2 nanotube sheets and used for monitoring gases such as for H_2, CO, and ethylene oxide [17]. Flexible three-dimensional SnO_2 nanoarrays were prepared on a CC using atomic layer deposition method [18]. The nanoscale photodetectors based on the flexible SnO_2 nanostructure on CC demonstrated excellent ultraviolet light selectivity, a high-speed response time less than 0.3 s, and dark current as low as 2.3 pA. A Periyakaruppan *et al.,* (2011) developed a carbon nanofiber based nanoelectrode array for the suitable detection of bio-threat agents. They reported that ricin detection using antibody and aptamer probes immobilized on a nanoelectrode array consisting of vertically aligned carbon nanofibers. The biosensor chips are fabricated on a wafer scale using steps common in integrated circuit manufacturing [19]. In 2014, Siwen Zhang *et al.,* described work on SnO_2 nanostructured successfully coated on CC by chemical vapor deposition method and used as flexible substrate. Further they analyzed structural, morphological and optical properties of SnO_2/CC [20]. Also, recently our group developed new approach for SnO_2 coating on carbon yarn and it was directly used as binder free electrode for the sensitive and selective detection of dopamine with the limit of detection of 53 nM [21].

In *chapter II*, hydrothermal process was used to grow uniform SnO_2 nanoflakes onto the CCY. These nanoflakes integrated SnO_2/CCY electrode was directly used as the binder free working electrode for constructing electrochemical sensor for cortisol, an important steroid hormone find wide verities of applications in healthcare. The SnO_2 coated fibers were used as an immobilization matrix as well as signal generating probe for binder free detection of cortisol. Antibodies specific for cortisol are immobilized onto the SnO_2 coated CCY using standard EDC/NHS protocol (details are provided in the experimental section). The electrochemical property of the prepared electrode was assessed by using CV and DPV techniques. The SnO_2/CCY immunoelectrode showed the better sensitivity of cortisol with wide linear range and lower detection limit. Also, the prepared immunoelectrode exhibited better selectivity for cortisol in the presence of high concentration of interfering compounds, which has potential applications in wearable sensor fields.

2.2 Materials and methods

2.2.1 Chemicals and reagents

Analytical grades of tin chloride (V) hydrate ($SnCl_4.5H_2O$), sodium hydroxide (NaOH), 1-Ethyl-3-(3-dimethylaminopropyl)carbodiimide (EDC), N-Hydroxysuccinimide (NHS) cortisol, progesterone, testosterone, corticosterone, cortisone, cholesterol and bovine serum albumin (BSA) were purchased from Sigma Aldrich. The monoclonal cortisol antibody (Anti-C_{mab}) (2330-4809) was procured from East Coast Bio. Bleached and scoured CCY with the density and diameter of 0.35 g/cm^3 and ~350 μm was purchased from Vinpro Tech, Hyderabad, India. 10 mM phosphate buffer saline (PBS) with different pH values were prepared using disodium hydrogen phosphate (Na_2HPO_4), sodium chloride (NaCl), potassium chloride (KCl) and potassium dihydrogen phosphate (KH_2PO_4). All aqueous solutions were prepared with double-distilled (DD) water.

2.2.2. Synthesis of SnO_2 nanoflakes and integration with conducting fiber

SnO_2 nanoflakes were grown on the surface of the conducting carbon yarn (CCY) by a facile hydrothermal method. In a typical process, stoichiometric composition of NaOH

(0.3 M) was added to an aqueous solution of SnCl$_4$.5H$_2$O (0.5 M) and stirred for 30 min to form homogeneous mixture. Following this, the solution mixture was transferred to a Teflon vial (65 mL). Prior to the synthesis, CCY was first cleaned by sonication in acetone, DD water and ethanol for 30 min respectively. Cleaned CCY was immersed in this solution, placed in a sealed autoclave and heated at 180 °C for 5 complete hrs. The resulting yarn was allowed to cool down to room temperature naturally and it was collected and rinsed with alcohol and DD water three times to remove the loosely attached products and residues on the surface. Finally, the yarn was dried at 60 °C overnight before any further characterization.

2.2.3 Growth mechanism of SnO$_2$ nanoflakes on CCY

The possible redox mechanism for the hydrothermal process of the SnO$_2$ nanoflakes formation is shown in Equation (Eq. 2.1 & 2.2),

$$SnCl_4.5H_2O + 4NaOH \rightarrow Sn(OH)_4 + 4NaCl + 5H_2O \qquad ----- (Eq.\,2.1)$$

$$Sn(OH)_4 \xrightarrow{\Delta} SnO_2 + 2H_2O \qquad ------(Eq.\,2.2)$$

During the hydrothermal process, the formation and grain growth of SnO$_2$ nanostructures onto the CCY is generally assumed to proceed through dissolution-recrystallization process. During the process hydroxides would dissolve in water and then re-precipitate as insoluble metal oxide particles [22]. The addition of NaOH with SnCl$_4$, the intermediate complex Sn(OH)$_4$ is precipitated at neutral pH. During the hydrothermal reaction, a large number of SnO$_2$ nanoparticles formed spontaneously from the dehydration of Sn(OH)$_4$. Free enthalpy of the system becomes negative as particle growth increases, owing to the gain in lattice energy to compensate the loss in surface energy [23]. The initial crystal nucleus began to develop as larger nanocrystals after being formed. As time increased, new crystal nuclei formed and developed as SnO$_2$ nanoflakes on the CCY [24, 25]. Here, the SnO$_2$ nanoflakes were formed without the addition of any surfactant or complexing agent.

2.2.4 Immobilization of Anti-C$_{mab}$ onto a SnO$_2$/CCY electrode

Covalent immobilization of monoclonal cortisol antibody (Anti-C$_{mab}$) was achieved via amide bond formation between an NH group of SnO$_2$ and a COOH group of Anti-C$_{mab}$

using EDC as the coupling agent and NHS as the activator. For binding, 70 µL of 2 µg/mL Anti-C_{mab} solution in PBS (10 mM, pH 7.0) containing 0.4 M EDC and 0.3 M NHS was poured onto the surface of SnO_2/CCY electrode and incubated for 120 mins in a humid chamber. The fabricated Anti-C_{mab}/SnO_2/CCY electrode was washed with PBS (10 mM, pH 7.0) to remove any unbound Anti-C_{mab}. Then the followed by 30 mins of incubation, the 40 µg/mL BSA solutions in PBS (10 mM, pH 7.0) for blocking of non-specific binding of SnO_2/CCY electrode. The fabricated BSA/Anti-C_{mab}/SnO_2/CCY immunoelectrodes were washed and stored at 4 °C when not in use [26, 27].

2.2.5 Sweat collections for real sample analysis

Sweat samples were collected immediately after 15-30 minutes of vigorous exercise, players and agriculture workers were the age group of 27-35. Sweat samples were collected in the morning and evening to examine whether sweat cortisol concentrations approximated the well-established theoretical value. For sweat collection, a cotton swab was rubbed over the scalp hair and neck, allowed to saturate and placed it in a 5 mL Eppendorf tube [28]. The collected samples were centrifuged for 5 mins and 1 mL of the supernatant was pipetted out and stored at -20 °C to maintain its biological activities. These samples were further used to detect cortisol using electrochemical immunosensor and the results were validated with commercial cortisol assay. The similar procedure has followed to the entire subsequent chapters for the real sample analysis. All these procedures were carried out as per the Departmental Ethics approval committee, Bharathiar University guidelines and regulations based on the approval of the Bharathiar University human ethical clearance committee.

2.2.6 Materials characterizations

Structural features of prepared nanostructures on CCY were investigated using Rigaku uttima IV X-ray diffractometer (using Cu Kα radiation at a wavelength of 1.5406 Å). The functional groups of the materials were identified by Bruker Tensor 27 Fourier transform infrared spectrometer (FT-IR) and Raman spectra were recorded using a Horiba Jobin-LabRam-HR system at 514 nm excitation. The morphologies were observed by field emission scanning electron microscopy (FESEM) on FEI Quanta-250 FEG microscope. The compositions of the materials were confirmed using energy dispersive X-ray spectrometry

(EDS) equipped with FESEM instrument. The high-resolution transmission electron microscopy (HRTEM) images were recorded on a JEM-2100FS instrument (JEOL) operating at 200 kV to further confirm the morphology of the samples. Surface area measurements were carried out using Brunauer-Emmett-Teller (BET) Quantachrome Nova 1200e (USA) instrument with N_2 as the analysis gas. The variation of electrical resistance of the prepared materials was monitored and recoded using Agilent B2902A source meter. The mechanical properties of the pristine and modified CCYs were examined using the universal testing machine (UTM) (Zwick Roell). The wettability nature of the fabricated electrodes was analysed using a contact angle meter (KRÜSS, DSA 20E) armed with a CCD camera module.

An *in vitro* Cytotoxicity test was performed for the prepared samples and analyzed as per ISO 10933:5. The L929 cells were procured form National Center for Cell Lines (NCCS) and the culture medium was replaced in fresh minimum essential medium (MEM). The cells were seeded at a concentration of 2×10^5 cells per well, in 200 µl of MEM supplemented with 10% FBS and allowed to attach for 4 hrs in 5% CO_2 incubator. Then sterilized test samples were placed in the cell culture media using a sterile forceps and further incubated for 24 hrs. After 24 hrs, 200 µL MTT (1 mg/mL) were slowly added in all the wells and incubated at 37 °C for 4 hrs. After the incubation, DMSO were added in the wells and read at 570 nm using Biotek multi-mode plate reader. Triplicates were performed for each test. The cell viability were calculated using the following formula

$$Cell\ viability = (Treated\ /\ Control)\ *\ 100$$

The means of the treatment group was compared with negative control using analysis of variance (ANOVA) followed by Dunnett's test using IBM SPSS software for windows, v.17 (IBM Corporation, Aramok, USA). Data represent as mean ± standard deviation (S.D) and probability level of P<0.01 were considered as statically significant. Data plotting and line fitting were carried out by Origin Pro-8 (Originlab, Northampton, MA, USA).

The conventional three-electrode electrochemical workstation (BioLogic SP-50) was used for all the experiment. In the cell, the prepared immunoelectrodes was used as the working electrode. A platinum wire and Ag/AgCl was used as the counter and reference electrodes, respectively.

The metal oxides used in present work, MWCNTs and MWCNT based hybrids integrated on CCY electrodes were all analyzed using these analytical techniques and results were discussed in their respective chapters.

2.3 Results and discussion

2.3.1 XRD analysis of CCY and SnO$_2$/CCY

Figure. 2.2 compares the powder XRD patterns of bare CCY and SnO$_2$ nanoflakes coated CCY. It was evident from Fig. 2.2, the pattern shows a broad diffraction peak of pure carbon yarn around at 26° and 43.2° that can be indexed to the (002) and (100) plane respectively which is the characteristic peaks of the carbon material [29, 30].

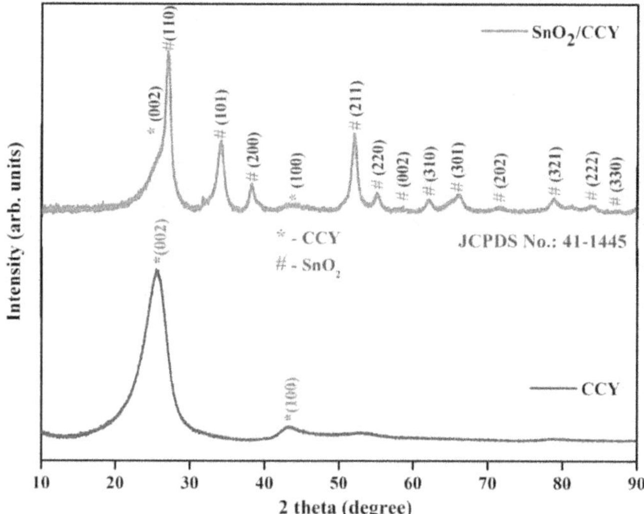

Fig. 2.2 X-ray diffraction patterns of CCY and SnO$_2$/CCY

All the diffraction peaks in Fig. 2.2 at 2θ values of 26.61, 33.89, 37.95, 51.78, 54.74, 61.82 and 65.79 were indexed to the tetragonal phase of SnO$_2$ on CCY with calculated lattice parameters of a = 4.738 and c = 3.187Å. The patterns are in good agreement with the reported values (JCPDS # 41-1445) [31], which confirmed the successful integration of SnO$_2$ on CCY. It is interesting to note that no distinct intense peaks related to carbon were observed after the integration of SnO$_2$ in the XRD results, this could be due to low crystallinity of carbon and adequate uniformity and thickness of the deposited SnO_2 nanoparticles onto the CCY surface. Apart from these, no other peaks were detected which implied that the absence of any impurities and that the fibers were composed of SnO_2 and carbon only. This is a clear indicator of a high purity of the SnO_2/CCY product.

The SnO_2 crystalline size on CCY was calculated as ~ 6 nm using Scherrer's formula mentioned below (Eq. 2.3) according to the diffraction peak of SnO_2 (101) plane,

$$D = k\lambda/\beta cos\theta \quad --------- \quad (Eq.\,2.3)$$

Where, K is a shape factor ($K = 0.9$), λ is 1.54056 Å, β is half peak width and θ is diffraction angle.

2.3.2 FT-IR spectra of CCY and SnO_2/CCY

The integration of SnO_2 onto the CCY was further investigated by FT-IR spectra and the results are shown in Fig. 2.3. The IR spectrum of CCY showed a characteristic peak at 1585 cm^{-1} corresponds to C=C bond. The stretching vibration peak observed at 1063 cm^{-1} is assigned to C-O-C bond and the peak at 1730 cm^{-1} corresponds to C=O group of carbon in the CCY. The absorption peaks at 2912 and 2849 cm^{-1} are due to C−H stretching. A strong absorption band at 3410 cm^{-1} corresponds to O-H stretching vibration and O-H deformation vibration peak at 1390 cm^{-1} observed due to small amounts of absorbed water. The presence of Sn–O–Sn symmetric stretching at 852 cm^{-1} and Sn–O asymmetric stretching at 577 cm^{-1} in SnO_2/CCY confirmed the presence of SnO_2 on the CCY [32].

Moreover, in the FT-IR spectrum of SnO_2/CCY, the C=C bond got shifted to lower wavenumber from 1585 cm^{-1} to 1562 cm^{-1} resultant from the interaction of Sn with carbon functional moieties. Further C=O vibration band shifted towards higher wavenumber from 1730 cm^{-1} to 1743 cm^{-1} due to the introduction of metal ion with subsequent reduction. The peak shift was due to the coverage of SnO_2 nanoflakes on CCY and it evidenced the successful deposition of SnO_2 on CCY.

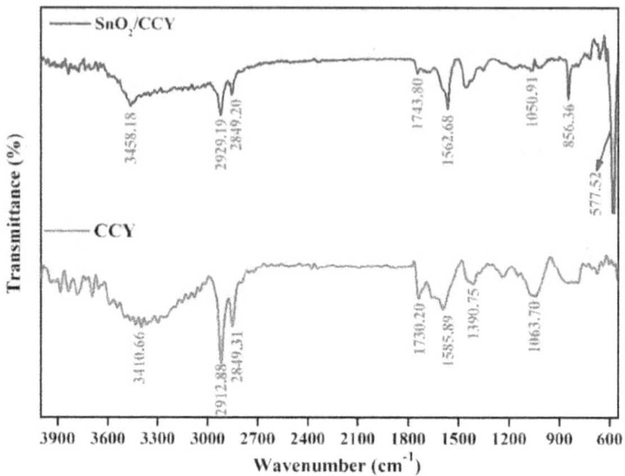

Fig. 2.3 FT-IR spectra of CCY and SnO₂/CCY

Additionally, a drastic decrease in the absorption of C=O, O-H (deformation, vibration) and C-O group from the SnO₂/CCY confirmed that most of the oxygen containing groups were removed from CCY [33]. The results were demonstrated that the successful integration of SnO₂ nanostructures on CCY.

2.3.3 Raman analysis of CCY and SnO₂/CCY

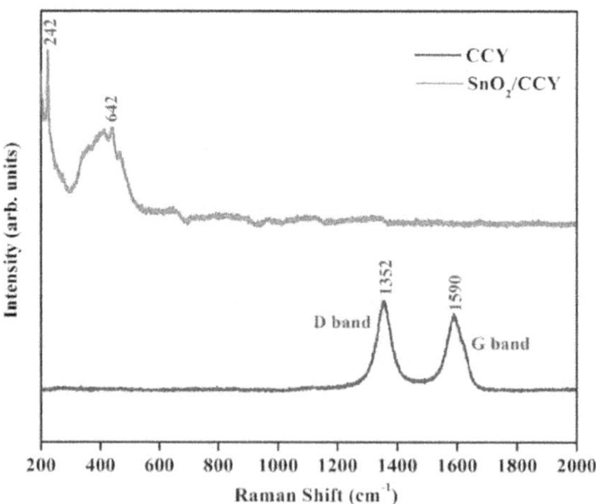

Fig. 2.4 Raman spectra of CCY and SnO₂/CCY

Raman spectroscopy is a vibrational technique highly sensitive to small changes in geometric structure and bonding. Hence, it is used widely to study the carbon materials. Raman spectra of the CCY and SnO_2/CCY nanoflakes are shown in Fig. 2.4. Two strong absorption peaks at 1352 and 1590 cm^{-1} corresponding to the D and G band respectively for CCY [34]. In the spectrum of SnO_2 on CCY, the bands located at 242 and 642 cm^{-1} could be attributed to active vibration modes of E_u and A_{1g} respectively, which originated from SnO_2 nanoflakes. These Raman bands are in good agreement with the tetragonal rutile phase of SnO_2 which was previously reported [35-37]. It is important to note the absence of impurity peaks in the spectrum of SnO_2/CCY which further confirmed the purity and uniform coating of SnO_2 on CCY via the hydrothermal process.

2.3.4 Morphological and compositional analysis of CCY and SnO_2/CCY

The morphology of the hydrothermally prepared SnO_2/CCY was analyzed using FE-SEM and depicted as in Fig. 2.5. The Fig. 2.5 (a) shows the morphology of pure CCY which consists of smaller fibers with a smooth surface. The inset showed the clearer picture of the smooth fiber. Fig. 2.5 (b-e) show the as-prepared SnO_2 integrated CCY at different magnifications. The nanoflakes network like structure was uniformly grown on the entire surface textile substrate of CCY. The SnO_2 have thin nanoflakes with a thickness of ~ 20 nm, and a height of approximately ~ 400 nm. After coating, the SnO_2 show a rough surface and have a larger diameter than pristine CCY (Fig. 2.5 d & e). Also, Fig. 2.5 (f) shows the coloring image of SnO_2/CCY.

The hydrothermal process was highly scalable, because this was performed in a solution media which regulates the rate and uniformity of nucleation, growth size, morphology and aggregation control that is not possible with many other synthesis processes. The interconnected construction of SnO_2 nanoflakes can significantly increase the electrolyte-accessible surface area on CCY and consequently enhance its electrochemical activity for cortisol oxidation.

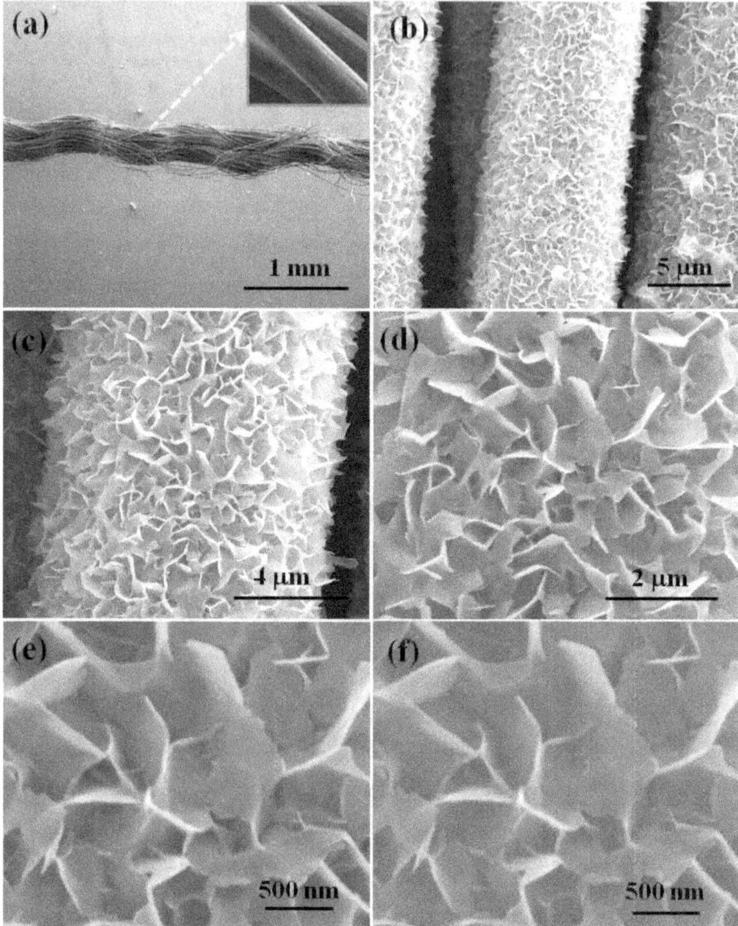

Fig. 2.5. FESEM images of (a) bare CCY, (b–e) SnO$_2$/CCY with different magnifications and (f) Coloring image

The EDS study was also performed for the chemical analysis of the SnO$_2$ nanoflakes integrated fibers (Fig. 2.6a). The EDS spectrum shows the peaks corresponding to Sn (45.86 wt. %), O (13.77 wt. %), C (44.27 wt. %). The chemical composition further confirmed by EDS mapping which evidenced (Fig. 2.6b) that SnO$_2$ is uniformly distributed over entire surface of CCY.

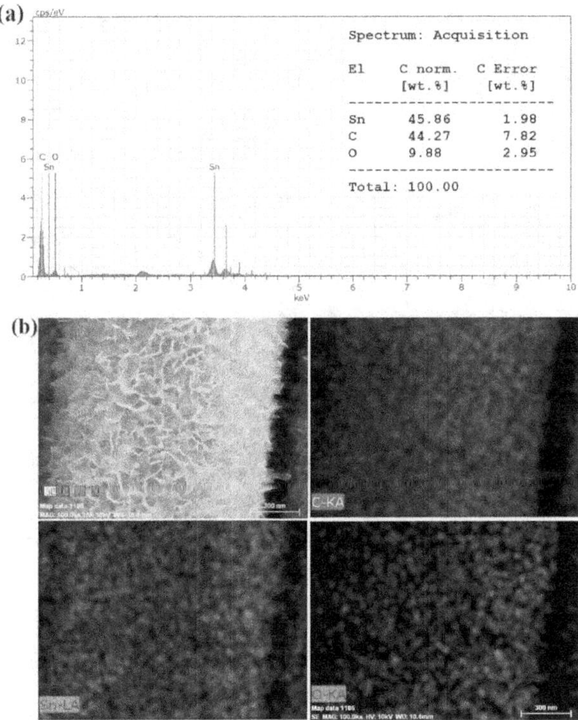

Fig. 2.6 (a) EDS spectra and (b) EDS mapping of SnO_2 /CCY

2.3.5 Electrical and mechanical properties of CCY and SnO_2/CCY

The electrical resistance of 5 cm long CCY and SnO_2 coated CCY was measured in order to investigate its electrical properties. The resistance of the SnO_2/CCY (68 ± 1.5 Ω) increased when compared to the untreated CCY (36 ± 1 Ω) and. B.S. Shim *et al.,* reported the reasonably low electrical resistance of yarn allows for suitable sensing applications that may not require any additional electronics or convertors [38]. Also, conductivity of SnO_2/CCY was demonstrated by powering an LED device connected to a battery as shown in Fig. 2.7. The average weight of SnO_2 was measured by checking the weight of CCY before and after SnO_2 hydrothermal deposition and the weight of 5 cm length CCY and SnO_2/CCY were 1.23 and 2.3 mg respectively.

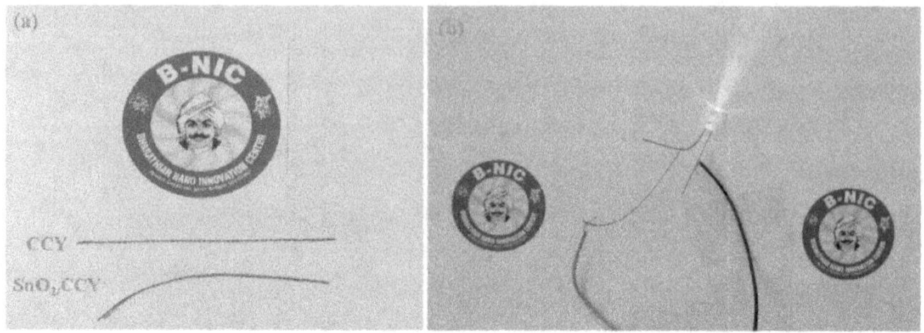

Fig. 2.7 Photographs of CCY–SnO₂/CCY; (a) Comparison of the pure CCY and SnO₂ Coated CCY (b) Demonstration of LED emission with the current passing through SnO₂ coated yarn

The mechanical property of the materials is one of the key issues for its use as a flexible electrode. In order to investigate the mechanical properties of CCY and SnO₂/CCY, the fiber electrodes were investigated for tensile, elongation and elastic modulus tests. The ultimate strength measured for SnO₂/CCY is found to be 31.86 MPa. This value is higher than that of untreated CCY (20.10 MPa). This implies that the strength of the fiber was improved when it is modified with SnO₂. Similarly, elongation and young's modulus of the SnO₂/CCY (6.82 % and 48.34 MPa) were improved after SnO₂ incorporation (7.53% and 37.17 MPa). The mechanical strength of the SnO₂/CCY is higher than that of the pure CCY due to a densification, and stronger adhesion of the fibers to each other by the material. The CCY became slightly harder after being coated with SnO₂ by hydrothermal method, yet it remained very flexible and soft which are more important features for the sensor applications.

2.3.6 Specific and assessable surface area of CCY and SnO₂/CCY electrode

The BET specific surface area of the CCY and SnO₂/CCY found to be 75.607 m²/g and 115.116 m²/g respectively. Clearly, well-defined network like SnO₂ nanoflakes on CCY possesses much higher specific surface area as compared to bare CCY. Generally, larger surface area means more active sites and diffusion pathways for ion exchange, which may lead to a larger response to the electrochemical cortisol detection.

Also, from the reversible redox reactions, the active surface area (A_e) value could be calculated using the standard Randle–Sevcik equation (Eq. 2.4) [39]. For this, we maintained a uniform fiber length of 5 cm throughout the experiments. Approximately 4 cm length fiber was soaked into the electrolyte solution.

$$i_p = 0.4463\, nFA_eC\sqrt{(\frac{nFvD}{RT})} \quad --------(Eq.\,2.4)$$

Where,

i_p = current maximum in amps; n is the number of electrons involved in the redox reaction; F = Faraday Constant in C mol^{-1}; A = electrode area in cm^2; D is the diffusion coefficient ($7.6 \times 10^{-6} cm^2 s^{-1}$), C is the concentration of the redox couple; v = Scan rate in mV/s; R = Gas constant in J K^{-1} M^{-1}; T = Temperature in K

The calculated value of A_e is 0.0700 and 0.0852 cm^2 for bare CCY and SnO$_2$/CCY working electrode respectively. It can be speculated that only part of the total surface area of the electrode is accessible for the electron – transfer on the SnO$_2$/CCY working electrode.

2.3.7 Wettability analysis of CCY and SnO$_2$/CCY electrode

Contact angle measurements are important to identify the hydrophilicity or hydrophobicity of the material surface for the wearable sensor applications. Often, when the contact angle is more than 90°, the material is considered to be a hydrophobic surface; otherwise, it is considered to be hydrophilic. The test liquid used was a 2.0 mL deionized water droplet under the ambient condition. In Fig. 2.8, an illustration is shown of the water droplets on the bare CCY surface in a static state at 145°. When compared to the unmodified CCY, the water droplet angle decreased to 47.1°. These observations suggested that the modifier results in the formation of a hydrophilic surface as a consequence of the hydrophilic functional group of the SnO$_2$/CCY (see FESEM images). The improved wettability would be attributed from the uniform hydrothermal growth of SnO$_2$ on CCY, as revealed by the FESEM images. The surface wettability can also supported the increased of loading of the active material [40, 41].

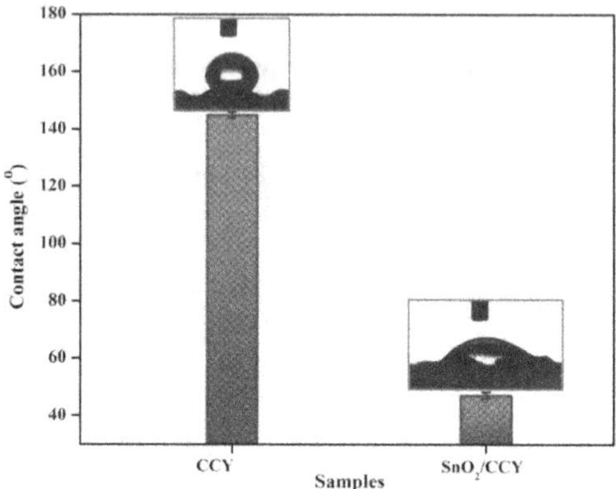

Fig. 2.8 Water contact angle of on CCY and SnO_2 modified CCY [Insets: The images of water contact angle]

2.4 Electrochemical analysis

2.4.1 Cyclic voltammetry studies

The stepwise preparation of SnO_2/CCY immunoelectrode and its functionalization for immunosensing has been studied using CV technique. The corresponding results are displayed in Fig 2.9. Bare CCY electrode (inset of Fig. 2.9) exhibited oxidation and reduction current magnitude in the range of 4 µA, which is typical for bare CCY electrode (curve: Black color). The magnitude of oxidation response current for SnO_2/CCY increases to 237 µA and only shows the peak for oxidation and reduction of SnO_2. The invisibility of CCY redox peaks due to the high intensity peaks for SnO_2, suggests the successful incorporation of SnO_2 nanoflakes on CCY with high concentration. The magnitude of the electrochemical current response was found to reduce as 172 µA after the immobilization of Anti-C_{mab} onto SnO_2/CCY nanocomposite electrode indicating the binding of Anti-C_{mab}. The decreased current response was due to hindrance in electron transport caused by the insulating nature of antibodies. Furthermore, the magnitude of current response of BSA/Anti-C_{mab}/SnO_2/CCY immunoelectrode was observed to be lower than that of Anti-C_{mab}/SnO_2/CCY electrode. Decrease in response current (~ 140 µA) was attributed due to the hindrance in charge transfer via insulating behavior of BSA blocked the non-specific binding cites on SnO_2/CCY.

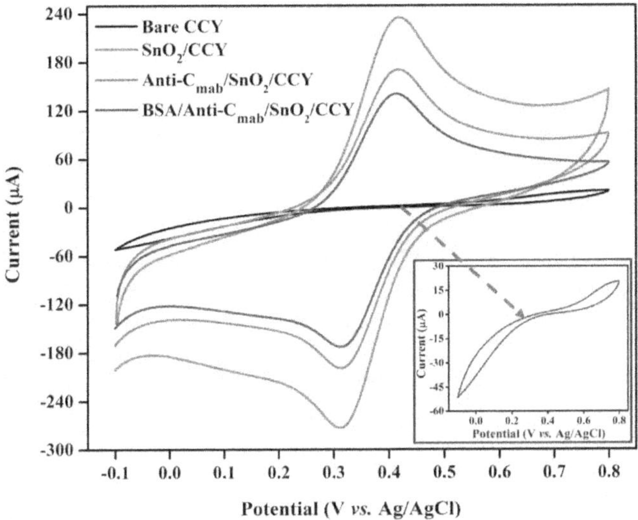

Fig. 2.9 CV analysis of step wise fabrication of BSA/Anti-C$_{mab}$/SnO$_2$/CCY immunoelectrode from CCY in PBS (10 mM, pH 7.0), [Inset: CV of bare CCY electrode]

2.4.2 Effect of pH

The sensing performance is dependent on electrochemical reaction of the immobilizing matrix and antibodies. In the immunosensors, the net charge and activity of amino acids available on antibody is responsible for antigen–antibody binding. Also, during immobilization, the proteins may lead to rearrangement and conformational changes in native structure. These features of antibody are known to depend on electrolyte pH, thus need to be optimized [27]. In Fig. 2.10a, it was observed that the magnitude of the electrochemical current response of BSA/Anti-C$_{mab}$/SnO$_2$/CCY immunoelectrode decreases while increasing pH from 5.5 to 6.5. Suddenly the oxidation peak current increased while pH 7.0, obtained maximum current. Again, increasing the pH up to 8.5 the peak current responses gradually decreased as shown in Fig. 2.10b. Because the immuno-electrode would have lost its electrochemical activity due to highly basic medium. So, the immunosensor response towards cortisol was found better in pH 7.0. Thus, pH 7.0 was chosen as the optimized working electrolyte pH. Moreover, the electrodes showed repeatable and reproducible electrochemical response behavior at pH 7.0.

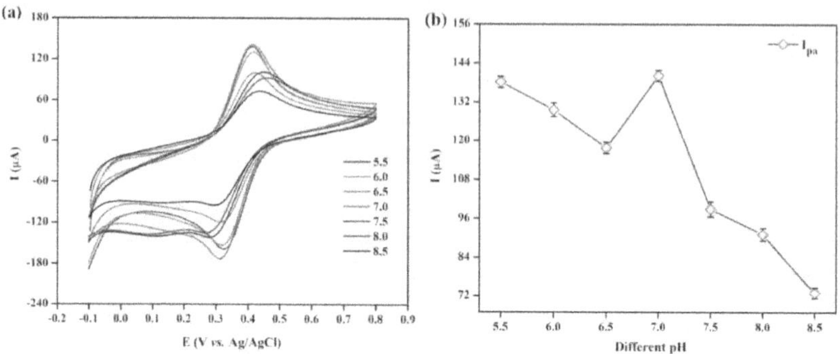

Fig. 2.10 (a) CV analysis of the BSA/Anti-C_mab/SnO₂/CCY immunoelectrode as a function of pH from 4.5 to 8.5 and (b) Linear plots of peak current *vs.* pH values

2.4.3 Effect of scan rate

In order to investigate the kinetics of SnO₂/CCY electrode in electrochemical reactions, the effect of different scan rates on the voltammetric response to cortisol were studied in detail.

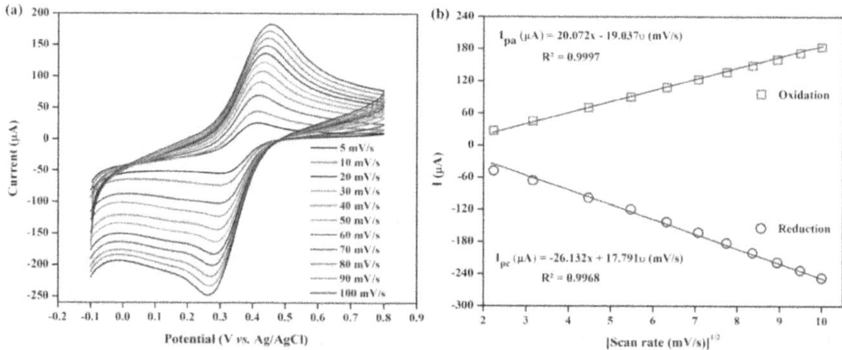

Fig. 2.11 (a) CV analysis of the BSA/Anti-C_mab/SnO₂/CCY immunoelectrode as a function of scan rates (5 to 100 mV/s) in PBS (10 mM, pH 7.0) and (b) Linear plot of the oxidation and reduction peak currents *vs.* square root of scan rates

Fig. 2.11a shows the scan rate responses of BSA/Anti-C_mab/SnO₂/CCY immunoelectrode at different scan rates ranging from 5 to 100 mV/s. It can be clearly seen from the Fig. 2.12a that both the anodic peak current (I_{pa}) and cathodic peak current (I_{pc}) of cortisol increased simultaneously while increasing the scan rate. Furthermore, I_{pa} and I_{pc} exhibited a linear relationship with a scan rate from 5 to 100 mV/s, which evident the electrochemical behavior of the cortisol was controlled by a typical surface-controlled process.

Moreover, both the I_{pa} and I_{pc} were linearly good scaled with the square root of scan rates ($v^{1/2}$) in the range of 5-100 mV/s as shown in Fig. 2.11b. The following equations (Eq. 2.5 and Eq 2.6) show the linear regression equation of I_{pa} and I_{pc},

$$I_{pa}(\mu A) = 20.072x - 19.037\upsilon\ (mV/s);\ R^2 = 0.9997 \qquad ------- (Eq.\,2.5)$$

$$I_{pc}(\mu A) = -26.132x - 17.791\upsilon\ (mV/s);\ R^2 = 0.9968 \qquad ------ (Eq.\,2.6)$$

The separation of peaks suggests that the process is not perfectly reversible; however, stable redox peak current and position during repeated scans at a particular scan rate suggests that composite based electrodes exhibit a quasi-reversible process.

2.4.4 Cortisol response studies of BSA/Anti-C_{mab}/SnO$_2$/CCY immunoelectrode by CV

The electrochemical current response of BSA/Anti-C_{mab}/SnO$_2$/CCY immunoelectrode has been studied using CV technique (Fig. 2.12) in triplet set using PBS (10 mM, pH 7.0) at scan rate 50 mV/s as a function of cortisol concentration ranging from 1 pg to 1 μg. All the immunoelectrodes were prepared in identical condition and displayed current value with a maximum variation of 2 %.

Fig. 2.12a depicts that the magnitude of electrochemical current response got decreased as a function of increment in cortisol concentration. Decrease in current response was attributed to the formation of insulating immunocomplex between Anti-C_{mab} and cortisol that hindered the electron transport. A calibration curve between the current response and logarithm of cortisol concentration has been plotted (in Fig. 2.12b), which reveals a linear correlation up to 1 μg and follow the equation of (Eq. 2.7),

$$\Delta I\ (\mu A) = -0.7647x + 125.06\ [Cortisol\ conc.\ (g/mL);\ R^2 = 0.9979 \qquad --- (Eq.\,2.7)$$

The immunosensor exhibited a linear detection range from 1 pg to 1 μg with a regression coefficient of 0.9979. The detection limit of the fabricated BSA/Anti-C_{mab}/SnO$_2$/CCY immunosensor is estimated as 4.5 pg using the following equation (Eq. 2.8)

$$3 * {SD}\big/_{S} \qquad - - - - \ - - - - - - - - - \ (Eq.\ 2.8)$$

Where, S is the slope of the calibration graph and

SD is the standard deviation of the baseline signal.

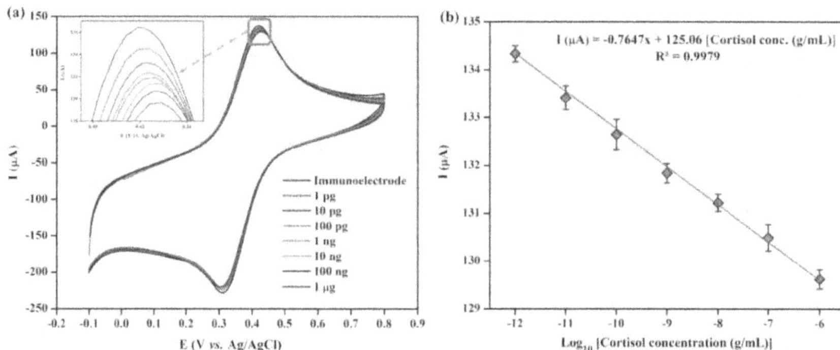

Fig. 2.12 (a) Electrochemical studies of BSA/Anti-C_{mab}/SnO$_2$/CCY immunoelectrode as a function of cortisol concentration varied from 1 pg to 1 µg in PBS (10 mM, pH 7.0) and (b) Linear plot between electrochemical peak current response and logarithm of cortisol concentration

2.4.5 Cortisol response studies of BSA/Anti-C_{mab}/SnO$_2$/CCY immunoelectrode by DPV

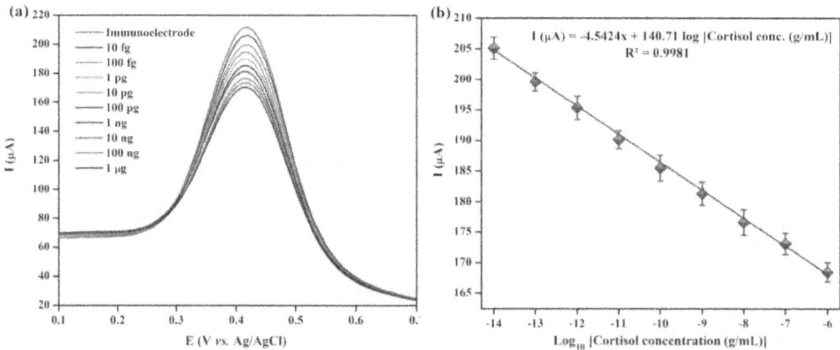

Fig. 2.13 (a) DPV analysis of the BSA/Anti-C_{mab}/SnO$_2$/CCY immunoelectrode as a function of cortisol concentration varied from 10 fg to 1 µg in PBS (10 mM, pH 7.0) and (b) Linear plot between electrochemical peak current response and logarithm of cortisol concentration

The electrochemical response of the BSA/Anti-C_{mab}/SnO$_2$/CCY immunoelectrode has been also studied as a function of cortisol concentration (Fig. 2.13) using the DPV method in PBS (10 mM, pH 7.0). DPV is a sensitive analytical technique to study electrochemical changes during biological reactions on the surface, mainly for signal amplification when the analyte concentration is very low [42]. All the measurements for cortisol detection at different concentrations were repeated three times using different electrodes. During the electrochemical response study, the magnitude of the electrochemical response current of the BSA/Anti-C_{mab}/SnO$_2$/CCY immunoelectrode was displayed to decrease on increasing the cortisol concentration (Fig. 2.13a). This confirms the successful formation of an immuno-complex between the antigen (Cortisol) and the antibody (Anti-C_{mab}). This resulted in a hindrance in electron transfer to the electrode due to the insulating behavior of cortisol. Figure 2.13b illustrated the linear calibration curve obtained between the logarithm of cortisol concentration and the magnitude of electrochemical response current exposed the good linear range from 10 fg to 1 µg with a correlation coefficient of 0.9981 followed the linear equation of Eq. 2.9,

$$\Delta I\ (\mu A) = -4.5424x + 140.71\ [Cortisol\ conc.\ (g/mL);\ R^2 = 0.9981\ -----(Eq.\ 2.9)$$

The detection limit of the fabricated BSA/Anti-C_{mab}/SnO$_2$/CCY immunosensor has been calculated as 1.6 fg using equation 2.7.

2.4.6 Interference studies

In order to evaluate the specificity of the prepared BSA/Anti-C_{mab}/SnO$_2$/CCY immunoelectrode have been tested 100 ng/mL of interfering substance, such as progesterone, testosterone, corticosterone, cortisone, cholesterol and BSA using CV technique in in PBS (10 mM, pH 7.0). The magnitude of current response for immunoelectrode was almost same, indicating that the fabricated BSA/Anti-C_{mab}/SnO$_2$/CCY immunoelectrode was specific and selective towards cortisol as given in Fig. 2.14. Though BSA, cholesterol and other derivatives of cortisol have been tested to indicate the specificity and selectivity of the prepared electrode, testing on biofluids such as sweat, serum and saliva were under way to validate the immunoelectrode for real application in cortisol detection [43].

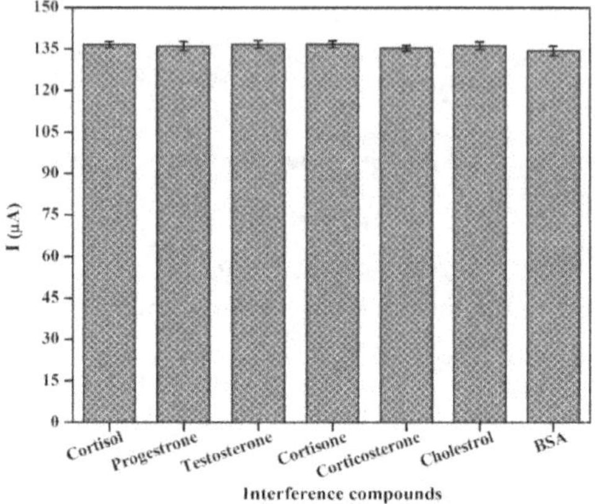

Fig. 2.14 Interference studies of BSA/Anti-C$_{mab}$/SnO$_2$/CCY immunoelectrode towards Progesterone, Testosterone, Cortisone, Corticosterone, Cholesterol and BSA with respect to cortisol (100 ng/mL) in PBS (10 mM, pH 7.0)

2.4.7 Stability, repeatability and reproducibility studies

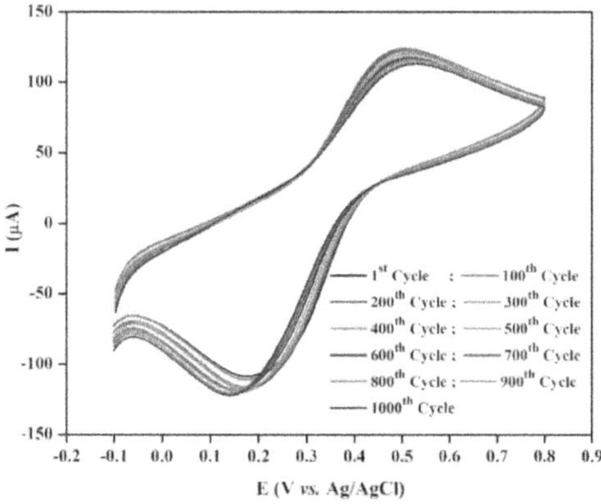

Fig. 2.15 The stability analysis of SnO$_2$/CCY immunoelectrode for 1000 cycles in 10 mM PBS

The stability of the SnO$_2$/CCY modified electrode was studied periodically towards the detection of 100 ng/mL of cortisol for four weeks. The BSA/Anti-C$_{mab}$/SnO$_2$/CCY immunoelectrode retains 95.4% of the initial current response of cortisol after the storage at 4 °C, which indicated that the modified electrode has a long-term life time or stability.

Also, the stability of SnO_2/CCY was investigated by measuring the current response using cyclic voltammetry for 1000 cycles in 10 mM PBS as shown in Fig 2.15. The RSD values were calculated from the current responses obtained for SnO_2/CCY of 2.15 % which indicating the good stability the fiber.

The relative standard deviation (RSD) of 2.2 % was found for 10 measurements of 100 ng/mL of cortisol by single SnO_2/CCY modified electrode. The five BSA/Anti-C_{mab}/SnO_2/CCY immunoelectrode were prepared independently and applied for cortisol detection to evaluate the inter-assay precision or the reproducibility of the modified electrode. The RSD of measurements was 3.2 % for cortisol, which was revealed the excellent reproducibility of binder free immunoelectrode. Thus, these results indicated the fabricated immunosensor has acceptable reproducibility and electrochemically stable for these biosensor applications.

2.4.8 Real sample analysis

We further examined the practicability of applying the immunosensor in clinical systems via analyzing several real sweat samples, and the results were compared with the commercially available chemiluminescence immunoassay (CLIA) sensing method which is given in Table 2.1.

CLIA is one of the widely used methods, currently being used in the laboratories to measure biological levels of hormones, drugs, vitamins, tumor markers, infectious disease markers, myocardial damage markers and autoantibodies. The sweat cortisol readings were validated using commercial chemiluminescence immunoassay (CLIA) kit purchased from Abbott Diagnostics (IL, USA). This is a competitive CLIA which uses polyclonal anticortisol antibodies.

Recommended assay protocols were followed to analyse salivary cortisol levels. In brief, sample and anti-cortisol coated magnetic microparticles are combined to create a reaction mixture. Cortisol present in the sample binds to the anti-cortisol coated microparticles. After incubation, cortisol acridinium-labeled conjugate was added to the reaction mixture. The cortisol acridinium-labeled conjugate competed for the available binding sites on the anti-cortisol coated microparticles. Following a second incubation, the microparticles are washed and pre-trigger and trigger solutions are added to the reaction mixture. The resulting chemiluminescent reaction was measured as relative light units (RLUs). A good correlation between the electrochemical measurements and CLIA results was observed. The results of both techniques are summarized in Table 2.1.

Table 2.1 Comparison of sweat cortisol estimated using chemiluminescence immunoassay and SnO_2/CCY based electrochemical immunosensor

Samples	CLIA method (ng/mL)	SnO_2/CCY immunosensor				
		Measured (ng/mL)*	Added (ng/mL)	Found (ng/mL)*	RSD (%)	Recovery (%)
1	34	32.14	50	81.32	2.283	99.02
2	47	43.62	50	94.81	3.423	101.27
3	41	41.69	50	94.38	3.064	102.93
4	68	65.83	50	114.96	4.253	99.24
5	25	24.67	50	75.69	3.563	101.36

*** The average value of three successive experiments**

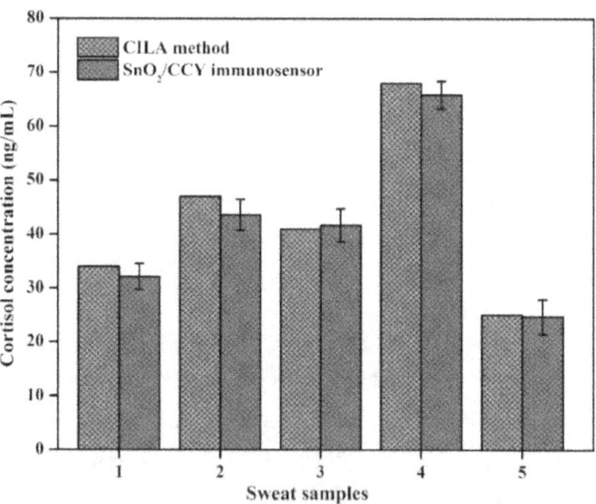

Fig. 2.16 Comparison graph of sweat cortisol estimated using chemiluminescence immunoassay and SnO_2/CCY based electrochemical immunosensor

Herein, CV method was used to detect the cortisol level in sweat. The RSD of the proposed immunosensor from 2.283 % to 4.253 % and the recovery rates of the samples ranged between 99.02 % and 102.93 %. The significant recovery percentages of cortisol in various sweat samples were determined. The outcome values were validated using commercially available CLIA sensing method as shown in Fig. 2.16.

2.5 Conclusions

In this chapter, hydrothermally derived network like SnO_2 nanoflakes on CCY were analyzed as a binder free immunoelectrode for the detection of cortisol. The prepared SnO_2 nanostructures possessed better physico-chemical properties compared to the previous literatures. But the electrochemical studies revealed a modest enhancement in its catalytic performance towards cortisol. This might result from low wettability surface features of SnO_2 were insufficient for enzyme loading and sweat based immunosensing analysis. In order to scrutinize the electrode performance we have attempt to prepare TiO_2, Fe_2O_3 and ZnO based on the variation in their redox behavior and the valuable outcomes were analyzed and discussed in subsequent chapters.

References

1. P. Sun, W. Zhao, Y. Cao, Y. Guan, Y. Sun, G. Lu, Porous SnO_2 hierarchical nanosheets: hydrothermal preparation, growth mechanism, and gas sensing properties, *CrystEngComm.*, **13** (2011) 3718-3724.

2. S. B. Patil, P. Patil, M. A. More, Acetone vapour sensing characteristics of cobalt doped SnO_2 thin films, *Sensor. Actuator B: Chem*, **125** (2007) 126–130.

3. V. Kumar, S. Sen, K.P. Muthe, N.K. Gaur, S.K. Gupta, J.V. Yakhmi, Copper doped SnO_2 nanowires as highly sensitive H_2S gas sensor, *Sensor. Actuator. B: Chem*, **138** (2009) 587–590.

4. R. Nurzulaikha, H.N. Lim, I. Harrison, S.S. Lim, A. Pandikumar, N.M. Huang, S.P. Lim, G.S.H. Thien, N. Yusoff, I. Ibrahim, Graphene/SnO_2 nanocomposite-modified electrode for electrochemicaldetection of dopamine, *Sens Biosensing Res.*, **5** (2015) 42–49.

5. C. Burda, X. Chen, R. Narayanan, M.A. El-Sayed, Chemistry and properties of nanocrystals of different shapes, *Chem. Rev.*, **105** (2005) 1025–1102.

6. M. H. Xu, F. S. Cai, J. Yin, Z. H. Yuan, L. J. Bie, Facile synthesis of highly ethanol sensitive SnO_2 nanosheets using homogeneous precipitation method, *Sens Actuators B Chem.*, **145** (2010) 875–878.

7. J. H. Lee, Gas sensors using hierarchical and hollow oxide nanostructures: overview, *Sens Actuators B Chem.*, **140** (2009) 319–336.

8. G. S. Pang, S. G. Chen, Y. Koltypin, A. Zaban, S. Feng, A. Gedanken, Controlling the particles size of calcined SnO_2 nanocrystals, *Nano Lett.*, **1** (2001) 723–726.

9. A. Gaber, M. A. A Rahim, Influence of calcination temperature on the porosity of SnO_2 by Co-Precipitation method, *Int. J. Electrochem. Sci.*, **9** (2013) 81-89.

10. H. Wang, J. Liang, H. Fan, B. Xi, M. Zhang, S. Xiong, Y. Zhu, Y. Qian, Synthesis and gas sensitivities of SnO_2 nanorods and hollow microspheres, *J. Solid State Chem.*, **181** (2008) 122–129.

11. M. N. A. Karlsson, K. Deppert, L.S. Karlsson, M. H. Magnusson, J. O. Malm, N. S. Srinivasan, Compaction of agglomerates of aerosol nanoparticles: a compilation of experimental data, *J. Nanopart Res.*, **7** (2005) 43–49.

12. N. Talebian and F. Jafarinezhad, Morphology-controlled synthesis of SnO_2 nanostructures using hydrothermal method and their photocatalytic applications, *Ceram. Int.*, **39** (2013) 8311-8317.

13. K. Ui, S. Kawamura, N. Kumagai, Fabrication of binder-free SnO_2 nanoparticle electrode for lithium secondary batteries by electrophoretic deposition method, *Electrochim Acta*, **76** (2012) 383–388.

14. Y. Zhang, Z. Hu, Y. Liang, Y. Yang, N. An, Z. Li, H. Wu, Growth of 3D SnO_2 nanosheets on carbon cloth as a binder-free electrode for Supercapacitors, *J. Mater. Chem. A*, **3** (2015) 15057–15067.

15. Q. Cheng, J. Tang, J. Ma, L. C. Qin, Polyaniline coated electro-etched carbon fiber cloth electrodes for supercapacitors, *J phy chem C.*, **115** (2011) 23584-23590.

16. Y. Liu, X. Fang, M. Ge, J. Rong, C. Shen, A. Zhang, H. A. Enaya, C. Zhou, SnO_2 coated carbon cloth with surface modification as Na-ion battery anode, *Nano Energy*, **16** (2015) 399–407.

17. J. Huang, N. Matsunaga, K. Shimanoe, N. Yamazoe, and T. Kunitake, Nanotubular SnO_2 Templated by Cellulose Fibers: Synthesis and Gas Sensing, *Chem. Mater.*, **17** (2005), 3513-3518.

18. K. Deng, H. Lu, Z. Shi, Q. Liu, L. Li, Flexible Three-Dimensional SnO_2 nanowire arrays: Atomic layer deposition-assisted synthesis, excellent photodetectors, and field emitters, *ACS Appl. Mater. Interfaces*, **5** (2013) 7845−7851.

19. A. Periyakaruppan, P. U. Arumugam, M. Meyyappan, J. E. Koehne, Detection of ricin using a carbon nanofiber based biosensor, *Biosens and Bioelectron*, **28** (2011) 428–433.

20. S. Zhang, B. Yin, Y. Jiao, Y. Liu, F. Qu, X. Wu, Nanosheet based SnO_2 assembles grown on a flexible substrate, *Appl. Surf. Sci.*, **305** (2014) 626–629.

21. S. Madhu, P. Manickam, M. Pierre, S. Bhansali, P. Nagamony, V. Chinnuswamy, Nanostructured SnO_2 integrated conductive fabrics as binder-free electrode for neurotransmitter detection. *Sens. Actuators, A*, **269** (2018) 401–411.

22. C. Guo, M. Cao, C. Hu, A novel and low-temperature hydrothermal synthesis of SnO_2 nanorods, *Inorg. Chem. Commun.*, **7** (2004) 929–931.

23. M. Niederberger, H.T Colfen, Oriented attachment and mesocrystals: Non-classical crystallization mechanisms based on nanoparticle assembly, *PhysChemChemPhys.*, **8** (2006) 3271–3287.

24. K. Jain, A. Shrivastava, R. Rashmi, Synthesis and controlling the morphology of SnO_2 nanocrystals via hydrothermal treatment, *ECS Trans.*, **1** (2006) 1-7.

25. T. Qi, Q. Wang, Y. Zhang, D. Wang, R. Yang, W. Zheng, Growth of flower-like SnO_2 crystal and performance as photoanode in dye-sensitized solar cells, *Mater. Des.*, **112** (2016) 436–441.

26. A. Dey, A. Kaushik, S. K. Arya, S. Bhansali, Mediator free highly sensitive polyaniline–gold hybrid nanocomposite based immunosensor for prostate-specific antigen (PSA) detection. *J. Mater. Chem.*, **22** (2012) 14763 – 14772.

27. S. K. Arya, A. Dey, S. Bhansali, Polyaniline protected gold nanoparticles-based mediator and label free electrochemical cortisol biosensor, *Biosens. Bioelectron.*, **28** (2011) 166–173.

28. E. Russell, G. Koren, M. Rieder, S. V. Uum, The detection of cortisol in human sweat: implications for measurement of cortisol in hair, *Ther Drug Monit.*, **36** (2014) 30-34.

29. S. He and W. Chen, Application of biomass-derived flexible carbon cloth coated withMnO_2 nanosheets in supercapacitors, *J Power Sources*, **294** (2015) 150-158.

30. J. Miao, F.X. Xiao, H.B. Yang, S.Y. Khoo, J. Chen, Z. Fan, Y. Hsu, H. M. Chen, H. Zhang, B. Liu, Hierarchical Ni-Mo-S nanosheets on carbon fiber cloth: A flexible electrode for efficient hydrogen generation in neutral electrolyte, *Sci. Adv.*, **1** (2015) 1-14.

31. H. Wang, F. Fu, F. Zhang, H. E. Wang, S. V. Kershaw, J. Xu, S. G. Sun, A. L. Rogach, Hydrothermal synthesis of hierarchical SnO_2 microspheres for gas sensing and lithium-ion batteries applications: Fluoride-mediated formation of solid and hollow structures, J. *Mater. Chem.,* **22** (2012) 2140–2148.

32. A. Kumar, L. Rout, R. S. Dhak, S. L. Samala, P. Dash, Design of a graphene oxide-SnO_2 nanocomposite with superior catalytic efficiency for the synthesis of b-enaminones and b-enaminoesters, *RSC Adv.,* **5** (2015) 39193 - 39204.

33. H. F. Ma, T. T. Chen, Y. Luo, F. Y. Kong, D. H. Fan, H. L. Fang, W. Wang, Electrochemical determination of dopamine using octahedral SnO_2 nanocrystals bound to reduced graphene oxide nanosheets, *Microchim. Acta,* **182** (2015) 2001–2007.

34. C. Zhang, P. Liang, X. Yang, Y. Jiang, Y. Bian, C. Chen, X. Zhang, X. Huang, Binder-free graphene and manganese oxide coated carbon felt anode for high performance microbial fuel cell, *Biosens Bioelectron.,* **81** (2016) 32–38.

35. J. X. Zhou, M. S. Zhang, J. M. Hong, Z. Yin, Raman spectroscopic and photoluminescence study of single-crystalline SnO_2 nanowires, *Solid State Commun.,* **138** (2006) 242-246.

36. C. S. Ferreira, P. L. Santos, J. A. Bonacin, R. R. Passos, L. A. Pocrifk, Rice Husk Reuse in the Preparation of SnO_2/SiO_2 Nanocomposite, *Mater. Res.,* **18** (2015) 639-643.

37. Y. Zhang, Z. Hu, Y. Liang, Y. Yang, N. An, Z. Li, H. Wu, Growth of 3D SnO_2 nanosheets on carbon cloth as a binder-free electrode for Supercapacitors, *J. Mater. Chem. A,* **3** (2015) 15057–15067.

38. B. S. Shim, W. Chen, C. Doty, C. Xu, N. A. Kotov, Smart Electronic Yarns and Wearable Fabrics for Human Biomonitoring made by Carbon Nanotube Coating with Polyelectrolytes, *Nano lett.,* **8** (2008) 4151-4157.

39. R. Thangaraj and A. S. Kumar, Graphitized mesoporous carbon modified glassy carbon electrode for selective sensing of xanthine, hypoxanthine and uric acid, *Anal. Methods,* **4** (2012) 2162–2171.

40. L. Zhang and H. Gong, A cheap and non-destructive approach to increase coverage/loading of hydrophilic hydroxideon hydrophobic carbon for lightweight and high-performance supercapacitors, *Sci Rep*, **5** (2015) 18108 (1-11).

41. D. J. Huang and T. S. Leu, Fabrication of high wettability gradient on copper substrate, *Appl Sur Sci.*, **280** (2013) 25–32.

42. R. Sriramprabha, M. Divagar, D. Mangalaraj, N. Ponpandian, C. Viswanathan, Formulation of SnO_2/graphene nanocomposite modified electrode for synergetic electrochemical detection of dopamine. *Adv. Mater. Lett.*, **6** (2015) 973-977.

43. B. Sun, Y. Gou, Y. Ma, X. Zheng, A. A. Abdelmoaty, F. Hu, R. Bai, Investigate electrochemical immunosensor of cortisol based on gold nanoparticles/magnetic functionalized reduced graphene oxide, *Biosens and Bioelectron.*, **88** (2017) 55–62.

Chapter III

TiO₂ Nanocubes Integrated Carbon Yarn as a Binder Free Electrode for Sweat Cortisol Measurement

Highlights

- A new attempt was made to grow highly-ordered TiO_2 nanocubes arrays directly on carbon fibers.

- Uniformly coated TiO_2/CCY was investigated as a binder-free electrode in cortisol detection.

- TiO_2/CCY immunosensor showed a low detection limit of 17 fg with wide detection range of 10 fg to 1 µg.

- For stress biomarker, TiO_2/CCY immunoelectrode exhibited better sensitivity, selectivity and long term stability.

Graphical illustration of immobilization and electrochemical immunosensing of cortisol on hydrothermally derived TiO₂ NRs/CCY with possible redox mechanism

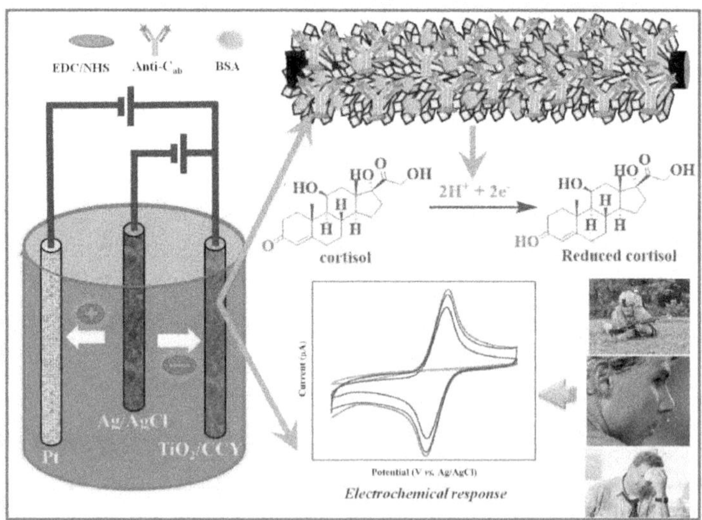

Electrochemical response

3.1 Introduction

Sensors have currently become gradually more important in a world where the technological advances require precise information of numerous categories [1, 2]. They have been extensively applied in the fields of environmental protection, medical diagnosis, industrial manufacturing, resources investigation and bioengineering [3-5]. Sensors can be made from a variety of materials depending on the functions they serve. High sensitivity, good selectivity and fast response are the general requirements for an excellent sensor. For large-scale applications, cost effective source materials and easy protection strategies are the prime criteria. With dramatic advances in nanotechnology, great progress has been made in recent years thanks to the newly developed nanomaterials in the field of sensor applications. Due to these inherent properties of nanomaterials, for example, small size and large surface volume ratio, they can amazingly improve the sensitivity of the sensors compared to bulk conventional materials [6-8].

One of the semiconductors, TiO_2 has received large attention since from 1972 when Fujishima and Honda discovered photocatalytic water splitting on a TiO_2 electrode under ultraviolet (UV) light [9, 10]. Over the past decades, TiO_2 has established applications in many promising areas ranging from photocatalysis, photovoltaic and sensors [11-16]. In addition to the above mentioned inherent advantages, TiO_2 nanostructured materials are nontoxic, biocompatible, photocorrosion resistive and cost-effective [17]. Moreover, the possible different morphological features enable them to achieve extraordinary large surface area along with unique chemical, physical and electronic properties [18, 19].

TiO_2 belongs to transition metal oxides family having three kinds of phase structures commonly found in nature: anatase (tetragonal), brookite (orthorhombic) and rutile (tetragonal) whose band gaps are 3.20, 3.02 and 2.96 eV, respectively. Anatase and rutile phases have wider applications because they are more stable than brookite structure [8, 10].

Rutile TiO_2 has a tetragonal structure which contains 6 atoms per unit cell (Fig. 3.1). The TiO_6 octahedron is slightly distorted and this rutile phase is stable at high temperature and pressures up to 60 Kbar, which is thermodynamically favorable phase [20-22]. However, Sclafani *et al.,* found that the rutile phase can be active or inactive, depending on its preparation conditions [23]. Zhang *et al.,* demonstrated that anatase and brookite structures transformed to the rutile phase after reaching a certain particle size, with the rutile phase becoming more stable than anatase [24]. The Anatase TiO_2 also has a tetragonal structure but the distortion of the TiO_6 octahedron is slightly larger when compared to rutile phase [25], as illustrated in Fig. 3.1. Muscat *et al.,* reported that the crystalline anatase and rutile phases of TiO_2 can be directly prepared using a hydrothermal method, the as-prepared TiO_2 appears to be amorphous and heat treatment has a crucial role in the phase transformation [26]. For example, with increasing the annealing temperature from 300 to 500 °C, amorphous structure can be changed into the anatase phase and further increment in the temperature up to 600– 700 °C, the anatase phase can be transformed into rutile phase [27]. In the practical applications, TiO_2 performance is commonly affected by the crystal phases, which can be attain through controlling their experimental conditions like preparation methods, pH, annealing time and temperature, etc. The rutile and anatase TiO_2 phases are the most preferred phases in the sensing applications [28].

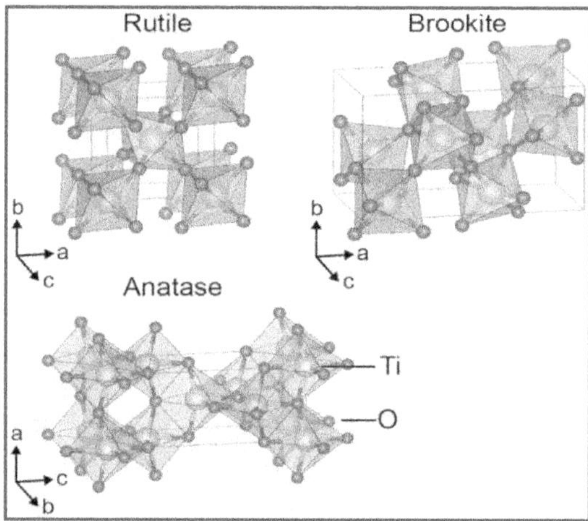

Fig. 3.1 Crystal structures of TiO_2 rutile (tetragonal), brookite (orthorhombic) and anatase (tetragonal) polymorphs

S. Liu *et al.,* have used the activated carbon fabric (ACF) as an additive free flexible substrate to grow TiO_2 nanosheets (TiO_2/ACF) due to its large surface area, high electrolyte adsorption capability and excellent mechanical flexibility. Combining the high pseudo capacitive TiO_2 with a strong ACF, with high tensile strength (12.7 MPa) found to be promising flexible electrode employed in LIBs. They have reported that TiO_2/ACF showed an exceptional high rate capacity of 97 mA h g^{-1} and superior long term cycling stability with a capacity of 130 mA h g^{-1} even after 2000 cycles [29].

S. J. Bao *et al.,* reported that uniform TiO_2 material was synthesized by a simple, CNTs-assisted hydrothermal method and was further investigated for protein immobilization and biosensing. The results demonstrated that the TiO_2 material has a large specific surface area and a unique nanostructure with a uniform pore-size distribution. Glucose oxidase immobilized on the material exhibited facile, direct electrochemistry and good electrocatalytic performance without any electron mediator. So they concluded that, TiO_2 is an attractive material for use in the fabrication of biosensors, particularly in enzymatic sensors [30]. Recently, J. Liu *et al.,* developed new strategy for achieving vertically-erected and hierarchical TiO_2 nanosheets arrays on carbon cloth as a binder free electrode for glucose sensing. The prepared protein impregnated mediator and binder free electrode showed a stable electrochemical response with good selectivity, high sensitivity (52 μA mM^{-1} cm^{-2}), low response time (<5 s) and low detection limit (23.4 μM) when compared to other reported literatures. The study suggested that the way for a promising strategy for preparing high-performance biosensors systems [31].

The active material of TiO_2 grown on conductive substrates, such as carbon fiber can effectively facilitate the electron transport and serve as the supporting matrix for antigen-antibody interactions. Moreover, such materials can be used as binder free flexible electrodes in wearable sensor devices, eliminate the use of polymer binder/conductive additives which used to limit the electrodes catalytic performances.

Recently our research group reported that the fabric based wearable biosensor for continuous monitoring of cortisol. In this, we used TiO_2 as active material for the preparation of binder free electrode on CCY for the detection of stress biomarker. Voltammteric measurement were performed in PBS at pH 7.0 to detect cortisol in the wide linear range of 50 pM to 350 nM with a detection limit of 10 pM. We suggested that the thread based sensor can be integrated with fabrics on a wearable platform to continuously monitor the cortisol levels in sweat [32].

In this *chapter III*, TiO_2 nanocubes have been grown on CCY using a facile hydrothermal method without the aid of sticky binders/additives. The as prepared TiO_2/CCY electrodes exhibited better electrocatalytic activity towards cortisol. The electrochemical responses via CV and DPV for the prepared TiO_2/CCY immunoelectrode towards analyte was resulted a wide linear detection range and lower detection limit. The TiO_2/CCY based immunosensor were tested with human sweat samples and the outcomes were validated with commercially available CILA method.

3.2 Materials and methods

3.2.1 Chemicals and reagents

Analytical grade of titanium tetraisopropoxide (TTIP) ($C_{12}H_{28}O_4Ti$), hydrochloric acid (HCl) were purchased from Sigma Aldrich). All other chemicals were purchased of analytical grade and used without further purification. All aqueous solutions were prepared using double distilled (DD) water.

3.2.2 Growth of TiO_2 nanocubes on conductive fiber

The TiO_2 nanocubes were anchored on CCY using a hydrothermal method according to the following protocol. 5 mL of HCl was added drop wise to an aqueous solution of TTIP (0.5 mL) and stirred for 30 min to form homogeneous mixture. Following this, the mixture was transferred into a Teflon vial (65 mL). The cleaned CCY fibers were immersed in this solution hanged in autoclave and heated at 180 °C for 12 hrs. The resulting yarns were allowed to cool down to room temperature naturally. The samples were collected and rinsed with alcohol and DD water three times to remove the loosely attached products and residues on the surface. The ordered nanocubes could be formed on CCY by calcining at 650 °C for 2 hrs to obtain stable rutile phase.

3.2.3 Growth and formation mechanism of TiO_2 nanocubes on CCY

E. Hosono *et al.*, and Z. L. Wang *et al.*, described the recrystalization process i.e. super saturation and growth process of TiO_2 nanostructures by hydrothermal method [33, 34]. The hydrolysis reaction in strong acidic media can be explained as follows (Eq. 3.1 – 3.3),

$$2Ti + 6HCl \rightarrow 2TiCl_3 + 3H_2 \qquad ---------- \qquad (Eq.\,3.1)$$

$$Ti^{3+} H_2O \rightarrow TiOH^{2+} + H^+ \qquad -------- \qquad (Eq.\,3.2)$$

$$Ti(OH)^{2+} + O_2^- \rightarrow Ti(IV) - oxo\ species + O_2^- \rightarrow TiO_2 \quad ---(Eq.\,3.3)$$

The proposed formation mechanism of TiO_2 nanocubes growth on CCY was as follows, Initially Ti species from TTIP precursor started to react with H^+ ions from concentrated HCl solution. It is well known that Ti^{3+} species are not stable in an aqueous solution, therefore $Ti(OH)^{2+}$ species were formed due to hydrolysis of Ti^{3+} species [35, 36]. According to the ''dissolve and grow method'', $TiOH^{2+}$ is oxidized to Ti(IV) by reaction with dissolved oxygen. The Ti(IV) oxo species is assumed to be an intermediate between TiO^{2+} and TiO_2, consisting of partly dehydrated polymeric Ti(IV) hydroxide [37]. The Ti(IV) complex ions were further used as the growth units on the carbon fiber surface [38].

For rutile TiO_2, a TiO_6 octahedron forms first by bonding of a titanium atom and six oxygen atoms. The TiO_6 octahedron then shares a pair of opposite edges with the next octahedron, forming a chain like structure. Because the growth rate of the different crystal faces depends on the numbers of corners and edges of the coordination polyhedra vacant, the growth of rutile nanocubes followed the sequence (110), (100), (101), (001). Thus, rutile TiO_2 nanocubes along [001] direction were formed [39, 40].

3.2.4 Fabrication of TiO_2/CCY based immunosensor

Covalent immobilization of Anti-C_{mab} was achieved between TiO_2/CCY using EDC and NHS as activator and coupling agent. For binding, 70 µL of Anti-C_{mab} solution containing 0.4 M EDC and 0.4 M NHS was poured onto the TiO_2/CCY electrode and incubated for 180 mins in a humid chamber. The fabricated Anti-C_{mab}/TiO_2/CCY electrode was washed with PBS, followed by 30 mins of incubation in 50 µL BSA solution for blocking the unbounded sites of Anti-C_{mab}. The fabricated BSA/Anti-C_{mab}/TiO_2/CCY immunoelectrode was washed and stored at 4 °C when not in use.

3.3 Results and discussion

3.3.1 XRD analysis of CCY and TiO_2/CCY

The XRD patterns of CCY and TiO_2/CCY are shown in Fig. 3.2. As can be seen, the XRD pattern of CCY showed two weak broad peaks at 26° and 43.2° corresponding to diffraction in the (002) plane and the (100) plane of aromatic layers of in carbon, which confirmed a predominantly amorphous structure present in the CCY substrate [41]. The XRD pattern of the TiO$_2$/CCY exhibited the characteristic diffraction peaks at $2\theta = 27.44°$, $36.08°$, $41.22°$, $44.05°$, $54.32°$, $56.64°$ and $69.08°$ corresponding to the indices (110), (101), (111), (210), (211), (220) and (301) respectively and the values are in good agreement with JCPDS data of rutile phase TiO$_2$ (JCPDS No.: 21-1276). This result proved that the successful formation of TiO$_2$ nanostructures on carbon fiber surface with high crystallinity and high purity [42].

Crystallite size was obtained using Scherrer's formula (Eq. 2.4). β selected diffraction peak corresponding to plane (101) and θ is the Bragg angle obtained from 2θ value corresponding to maximum intensity peak in XRD pattern (Fig. 3.2). The crystallite size obtained was ~5.6 nm.

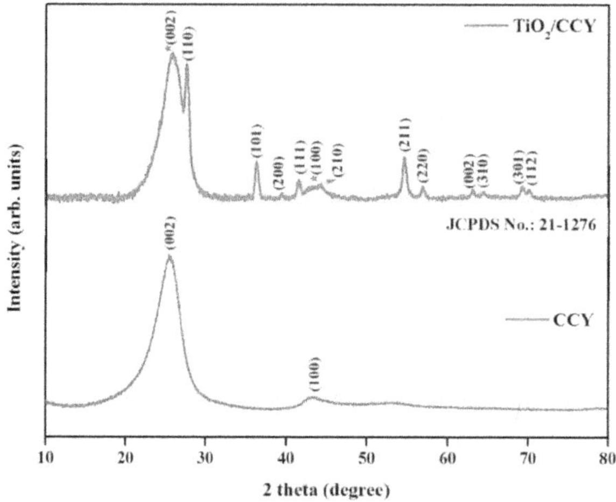

Fig. 3.2 X-ray diffraction patterns of CCY and TiO$_2$/CCY

3.3.2 FT-IR spectra of CCY and TiO$_2$/CCY

Figure 3.3 shows the FT-IR spectra of the CCY and TiO$_2$/CCY fibers. For the original CCY fiber, the characteristic peaks obtained at 3410 and 1390 cm^{-1} are assigned to the O–H stretching and deformation vibration, which attributed from small amount of absorbed water and residue from the pre treatment of CCY. The stretching vibration peak observed at 1063 cm^{-1} was assigned to C-O-C bond and the peak at 1730 cm^{-1}

corresponding to C=O group of carbon in the CCY. The absorption peaks at 2912 and 2849 cm^{-1} were referred to the in-plane bending of C–H. A sharp absorption peak at approximately 572 cm^{-1} could be assigned to the Ti-O stretching vibration. The peak corresponding peaks were assigned for the formation of TiO_2 nanocubes as shown in Fig. 3.3 (inset) [45]. No other new peaks appeared in the FT-IR spectrum of the TiO_2/CCY, which proved that a physical interaction caused the formation of TiO_2 nanocubes on CCY surface. Additionally, a significant decrement in the absorption of C=O, O-H (deformation, vibration) and C-O group from the TiO_2/CCY confirmed that most of the oxygen containing groups were removed from CCY [44]. The results were confirmed that the successful incorporation of TiO_2 nanostructures on CCY.

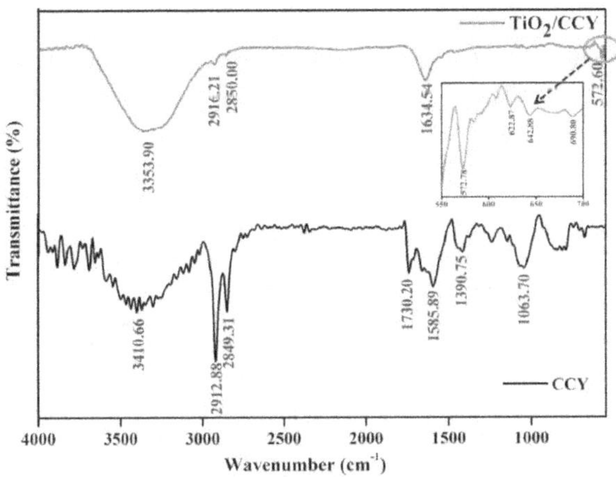

Fig. 3.3 FT-IR spectra of CCY and TiO_2/CCY

3.3.3 Raman spectra of CCY and TiO_2/CCY

Raman spectra were also recorded to analyze the functional properties and degree of crystallinity of carbon which is shown in Fig. 3.4. The broad characteristic peaks at approximately 1358 and approximately 1597 cm^{-1} arouse due to the presence of D band (disordered carbon) and G band (graphitic carbon), respectively. The intensity ratio of D and G bands (I_D/I_G) is about 1.19, which revealed the carbon fibers have been partially graphitized [45]. Compared with pure carbon yarn, the Raman spectra of TiO_2/CCY also clearly exhibited characteristic peaks at 143, 237, 321, 447 and 612 cm^{-1}, which could be assigned to the B_{1g}, E_g and A_{1g} respectively. Positions and intensity of the four Raman active modes could be well attributed to the rutile phase TiO_2 reference values. Rutile TiO_2 is tetragonal and belongs to $D_{4h}^{14}(P4_2/mnn)$ space group symmetry [46, 47]. Interestingly, a decrease in the intensity peaks of carbon was observed in the TiO_2/CCY spectrum which implied a tight integration of TiO_2 nanocubes on CCY. No impurity peaks were detected in these Raman spectra which ensured the purity of the prepared samples.

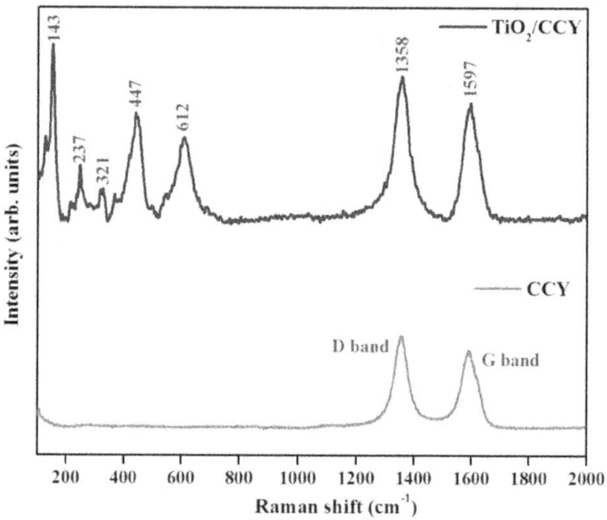

Fig. 3.4 Raman spectra of CCY and TiO_2/CCY

3.3.4 Morphological and compositional analysis of CCY and TiO_2/CCY

The microstructure and morphology of the one step synthesized TiO_2/CCY were examined using FESEM analysis. The image clearly revealed that the carbon yarn composed of small fibers with smooth surface as shown in Fig 3.5a. To determine the morphology of the obtained material, their low-magnification and closely magnified FESEM images were taken and exposed in Fig. 3.5(b-f). The FESEM image in Fig. 3.5b verified an over view morphology of a single carbon fiber encapsulated by fine and delicate TiO_2 nanocubes. TiO_2 nanocubes were distributed on the carbon fiber substrate in a uniform, highly ordered manner. The separated TiO_2 nanocubes could clearly found, and their average diameter was in the range from 50 to 70 nm. These intricate nanostructures of TiO$_2$ nanocubes potentially yielded extensive interface large active centers for the antigen and antibody interactions for the enzyme molecules.

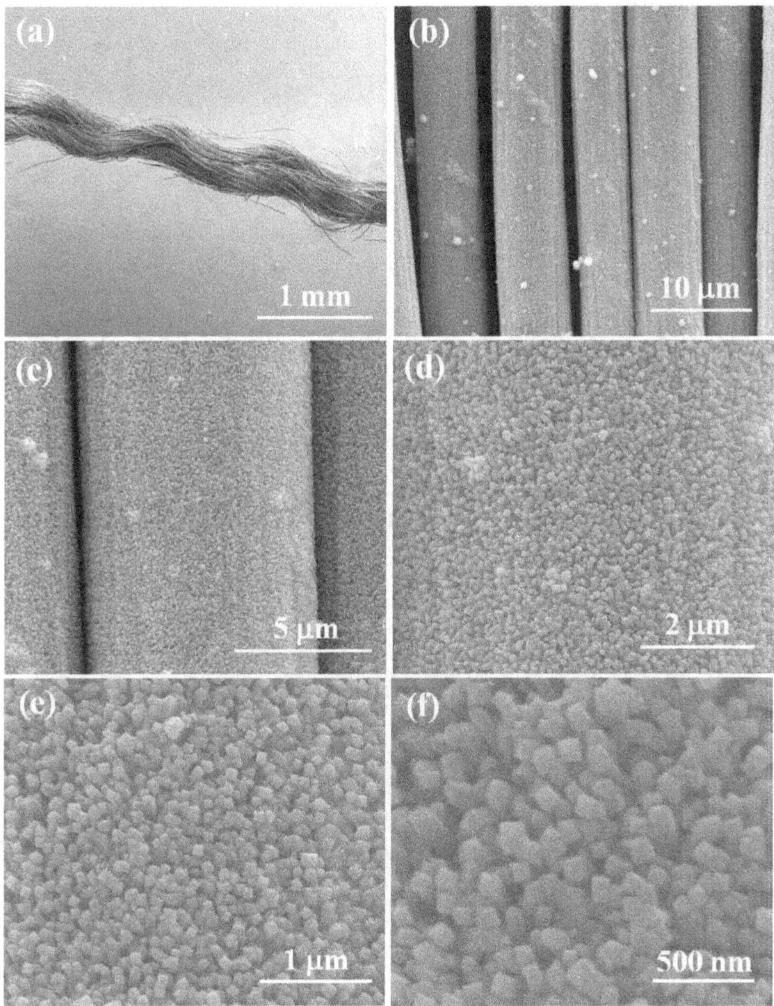

Fig. 3.5 FESEM images of (a) bare CCY and (b-f) TiO$_2$/CCY with different magnifications

The above EDS spectrum expressed the peaks corresponding to Ti (43.80 wt. %), O (18.12 wt. %) and C (38.08 wt. %) as given in Fig. 3.6a (Insert: Table). The absence of impurities peaks confirmed the presence, integration and purity of TiO_2 into the CCY. Elemental mappings of TiO_2/CCY fiber revealed that Ti, O and C were uniformly distributed on CCY (Fig. 3.6b).

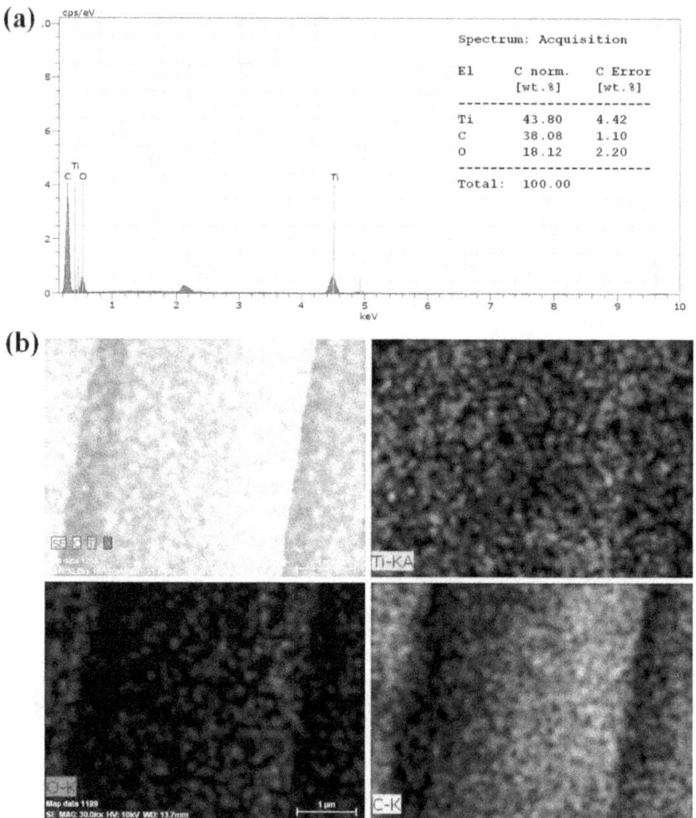

Fig. 3.6 (a) EDS spectra and (b) EDS mapping of TiO_2/CCY

3.3.6 Electrical and mechanical properties of CCY and TiO_2/CCY

To examine the electrical resistance of CCY and TiO_2 coated CCY, the 5 cm long yarn was used and measured. The current resistance of the TiO_2/CCY (63.4±1.8 Ω)

increased when compared to the uncoated bare CCY (36 ±1 Ω). Also, conductivity of TiO2/CCY was demonstrated by powering an LED device connected to a battery as shown in Fig. 3.7. The average weight of TiO2 was measured by checking the weight of CCY before and after TiO2 nanocubes hydrothermal deposition and the weight of 5 cm length CCY and TiO2/CCY were found as 1.22 and 2.2 mg respectively.

In order to investigate the mechanical properties of CCY and TiO2/CCY, the fiber electrodes were investigated for hardness, elastic modulus and elongation. The ultimate strength measured for TiO2/CCY is found to be 28.46 MPa. This value was higher than that of untreated CCY (20.10 MPa). This implied that the strength of the fiber was improved when it is integrated with TiO2. Similarly, elongation and young's modulus of the TiO2/CCY (5.46 % and 42.56 MPa) were improved after TiO2 incorporation (7.53% and 42.56 MPa). The mechanical strength of the TiO2/CCY was higher than that of the pure CCY due to the uniform and thickness coating of TiO2 nanocubes on the CCY surface.

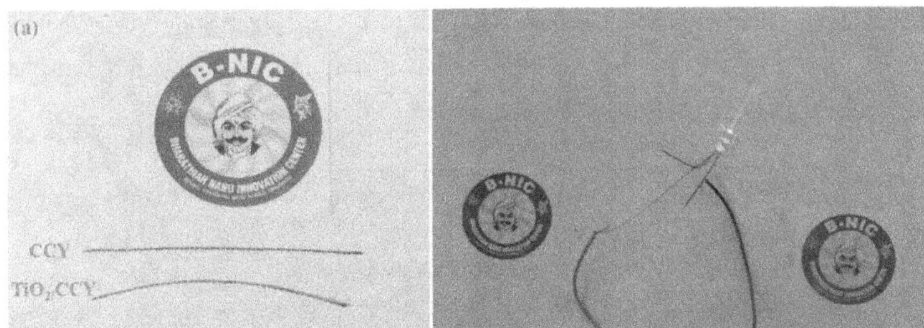

Fig. 3.7 Photographs of CCY-TiO2/CCY; (a) Comparison of the pure CCY and TiO2 coated CCY (b) Demonstration of LED emission with the current passing through TiO2 coated yarn

3.3.7 Specific and assessable surface area of CCY and TiO2/CCY electrode

The BET adsorption analysis showed that the specific surface area of TiO2/CCY is 108.48 m^2 g^{-1}. In TiO2/CCY, TiO2 nanocubes possessed higher specific surface area as compared to bare CCY. The high surface area can facilitate the diffusion pathway and adsorption of reactant molecules, resulting in a more efficient catalytic process in their sensor applications.

The assessable surface area of bare CCY and TiO$_2$/CCY were calculated. For this purpose, CV results were recorded for 2 mM [K$_3$Fe(CN)$_6$] using 10 mM PBS as the supporting electrolyte at different scan rates. Well-defined redox couple was observed for TiO$_2$/CCY electrode due to the presence of Fe^{3+}/Fe^{2+}. For a reversible process, the standard Randle–Sevcik equation (Eq. 2.3) applied. The slope of i$_p$ versus $\upsilon^{1/2}$ plot was then used to calculate the active surface area (Ae) of bare CCY and TiO$_2$/CCY and the determined values were 0.0702 cm^2 and 0.0894 cm^2, respectively. Thus, it was evident the effective working area was higher for the TiO$_2$/CCY compared to bare CCY.

3.3.8 Wettability analysis of CCY and TiO$_2$/CCY electrode

Contact angle measurements are important to characterize the hydrophilicity or hydrophobicity of a material surface. In Fig. 3.8, a graph is shown of the water droplets of the unmodified CCY surface in a static state (~150°). When compared to the unmodified CCY, the water droplet absorbed on the TiO$_2$ nanocubes coated CCY surface quickly which resulted in the decrement in angle with time (0°). These observations suggested that the modifier (TiO$_2$/CCY) consisted in the formation of a superhydrophilic surface which can be employed in non-invasive wearable sensors.

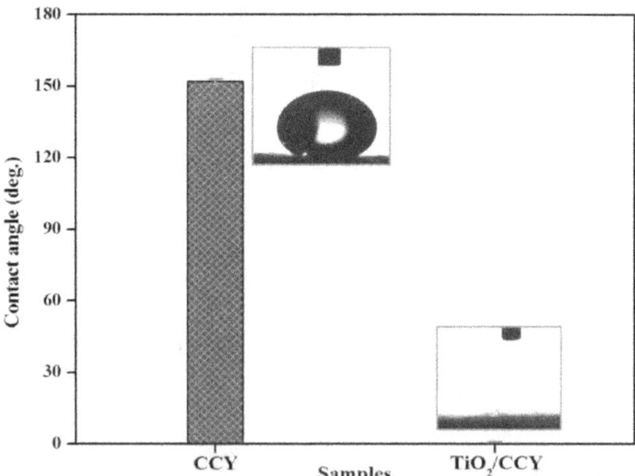

Fig. 3.8 Water contact angle of on CCY and TiO$_2$ nanocubes CCY [Insets: The images of water droplet with contact angle]

3.4 Electrochemical analysis

3.4.1 Cyclic voltammetry studies

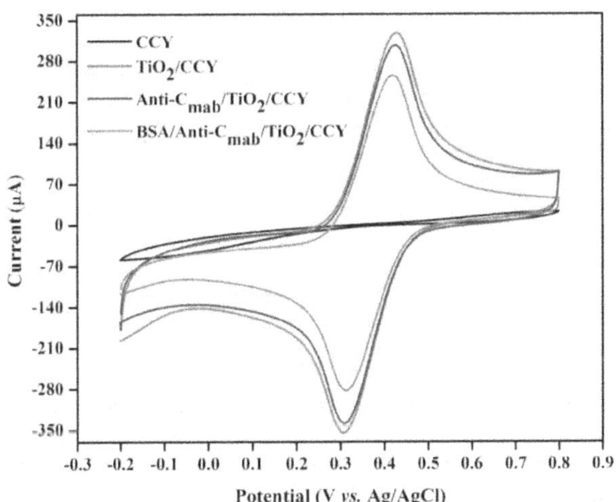

Fig. 3.9 CV analysis of step wise fabrication of BSA/Anti-C$_{mab}$/TiO$_2$/CCY immunoelectrode from CCY in PBS (10 mM, pH 7.0)

The stepwise assembly of the immunosensor was characterized by CV technique and the results are shown in Fig. 3.9. For this, electrochemical parameters were fixed as 10 mM PBS (pH 7.0) at 50 mV/s with the working potential range of -0.2 - 0.8 V. No anodic and cathodic peak current responses were observed for the bare CCY electrode. While the CCY electrode was modified with TiO$_2$ nanocubes, the magnitude of redox peak current increased ($\sim$ 330 µA) due to the active redox sites of TiO$_2$ on CCY surface. The electrochemical response current magnitude of Anti-C$_{mab}$/TiO$_2$/CCY decreased ($\sim$ 302 µA) after immobilizing the Anti-C$_{mab}$ via amide bond of NHS and EDC. The presence of insulating natured Anti-C$_{mab}$ on the surface hindered the electron transport, which confirmed the immobilization. The non-binding sites of the Anti-C$_{mab}$/TiO$_2$/CCY immunoelectrode were blocked using BSA. This also further decreased the electrochemical response ($\sim$ 256 µA), due to an oxidation and reduction in electron transport from electrolytes to the immunoelectrode. The developed BSA/Anti-C$_{mab}$/TiO$_2$/CCY immunoelectrode was subjected to further electrochemical characterizations.

3.4.2 Effect of pH

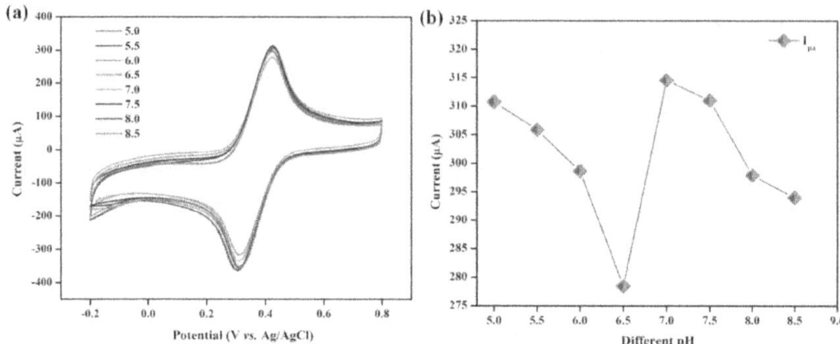

Fig. 3.10 (a) CV analysis of the BSA/Anti-C$_{mab}$/TiO$_2$/CCY immunoelectrode as a function of pH from 5.0 to 8.5 in PBS and (b) Linear plots of peak current *vs.* pH values

The influence of the pH of supporting electrolyte is another critical parameter for analyzing the electrochemical performance of the immunosensor which is shown in Fig. 3.10. Since the acidity of the solution significantly affects the redox behavior of the immobilized antibodies. Therefore, we analyzed and found that the magnitude of electrochemical response current of BSA/Anti-C$_{mab}$/TiO$_2$/CCY immunoelectrode decreased while increasing pH from 5.0 to 6.5. However, further increasing the pH to 7.0, the magnitude of the current was suddenly increased and showed a maximum response. Beyond increasing the pH upto 8.5 the current was gradually decreased. The maximum current was observed at the pH range of 7.0 -7.5. The corresponding linear plot of the pH values *vs.* oxidation peak current was given in Fig. 3.10b. From the outcomes, pH 7.0 was designated as the optimized working electrolyte because of physiological conditions [48].

3.4.3 Effect of scan rate

The scan rate (5-100 mV/s) dependent CV study was performed for BSA/Anti-C$_{mab}$/TiO$_2$/CCY immunoelectrode. A linear relationship between the magnitude of electrochemical response current and the square root of the scan rate was observed as shown in Fig. 3.11a and b. The linear relationship equation follows (Eq. 3.4 & 3.5),

$$I_{pa}(\mu A) = 41.183x - 64.50\upsilon \ (mV/s); \ R^2 = 0.999 \quad ------(Eq.\,3.4)$$

$$I_{pc}(\mu A) = -40.006x + 19.708\upsilon \ (mV/s); \ R^2 = 0.998 \quad ----- (Eq.\,3.5)$$

The observed well-defined stable redox peaks as a function of scan rate suggested that was a surface-controlled electrochemical process. Further, stable redox peak current and position during repeated scans at a particular scan rate implied that the developed electrodes exhibited a quasi-reversible process.

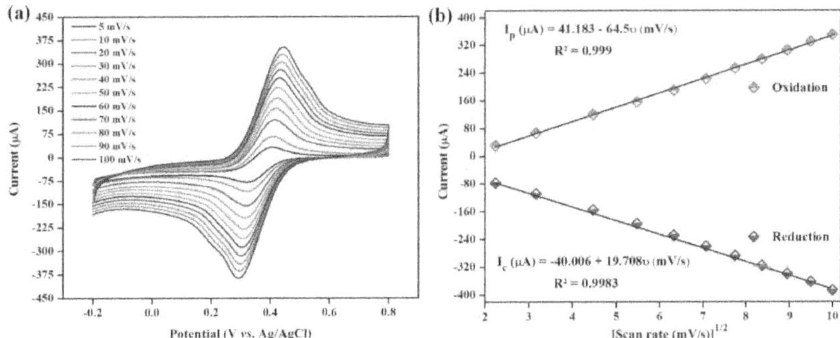

Fig. 3.11 (a) CV analysis of the BSA/Anti-C$_{mab}$/TiO$_2$/CCY immunoelectrode as a function of scan rates (5 -100 mV/s) in PBS (10 mM, pH 7.0) and (b) Linear plot of the oxidation and reduction peak currents *vs.* square root of scan rates

3.4.4 Cortisol response studies of BSA/Anti-C$_{mab}$/TiO$_2$/CCY immunoelectrode by CV

The electrochemical response of BSA/Anti-C$_{mab}$/TiO$_2$/CCY immunoelectrode has been studied using CV method. The experiment was repeated in the triplet set using PBS at the scan rate of 50 mV/s as a function of cortisol concentration ranging from 10 fg to1 µg.

Figure 3.12a illustrated that the magnitude of electrochemical current response decreased while increasing the cortisol concentration. The decreased in response current endorsed the formation of insulating immune complex between Anti-C$_{mab}$ and cortisol that hindered electron transport. A calibration curve between the magnitude of oxidation peak current response and logarithmic concentration of cortisol were plotted (Fig. 3.12b), which revealed that the linear correlation upto 1 µg and corresponding equation is given below (Eq. 3.6),

$$\Delta I \ (\mu A) = -0.1702x + 250.86 \ [Cortisol \ conc. \ (g/mL); \ R^2 = 0.9987 \ --(Eq.\,3.6)$$

The prepared immunosensor exhibited wide linear range from 10 fg to 1 µg with a regression coefficient of 0.999. The detection limit of the BSA/Anti-C_{mab}/TiO$_2$/CCY immunosensor was calculated as 17 fg using standard equation (Eq. 2.8).

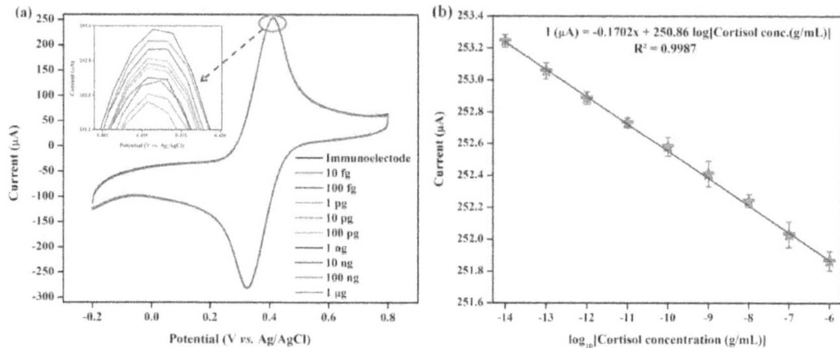

Fig. 3.12   (a) Electrochemical studies of BSA/Anti-C_{mab}/TiO$_2$/CCY immunoelectrode as a function of cortisol concentration varied from 10 fg to 1 µg in PBS (10 mM, pH 7.0) and (b) Linear plot between electrochemical peak current response and logarithm of cortisol concentration

3.4.5 Cortisol response studies of BSA/Anti-C_{mab}/TiO$_2$/CCY immunoelectrode by DPV

The electrochemical response studies were conducted using DPV sensitive technique. A standard successive addition method showed that the magnitude of response current decreased with increasing cortisol concentrations (10 fg - 1 µM) which is given in (Fig. 3.13a). This is due to the formation of immuno complexes between Anti-C_{mab} and cortisol resulting in electron charge transfer hindrance at the electrode electrolyte interface. The variation in electrochemical response current of BSA/Anti-C_{mab}/TiO$_2$/CCY immunoelectrode was linearly dependent to the logarithm of cortisol concentration (Fig. 3.13b) and obeyed the following equation (Eq. 3.7)

$$\Delta I\ (\mu A) = -0.7014x + 314.15\ [Cortisol\ conc.\ (g/mL);\ R^2 = 0.9962\ --(Eq.\,3.7)$$

The BSA/Anti-C_{mab}/TiO$_2$/CCY immunoelectrode exhibited wide linear range from 10 fg - 1 µg with a detection limit of 6.16 fg and a correlation coefficient of 0.9962.

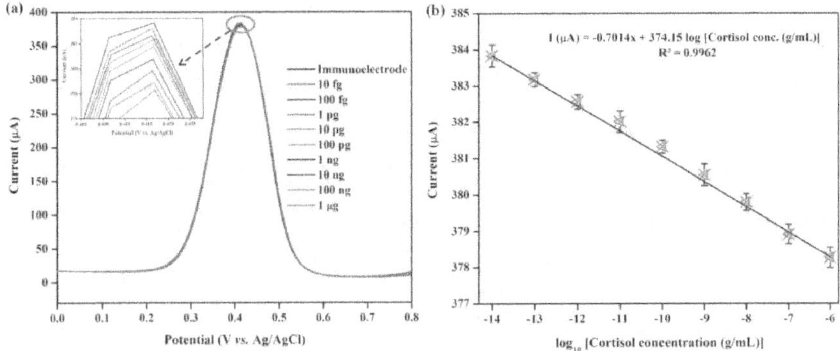

Fig. 3.13 (a) DPV analysis of the BSA/Anti-C$_{mab}$/TiO$_2$/CCY immunoelectrode as a function of cortisol concentration varied from 10 fg to 1μg in PBS (10 mM, pH 7.0) and (b) Linear plot between electrochemical peak current response and logarithm of cortisol concentration

3.4.6 Interference studies

Specificity is an essential analytical parameter which also influences the efficacy of an immunosensor in clinical applications.

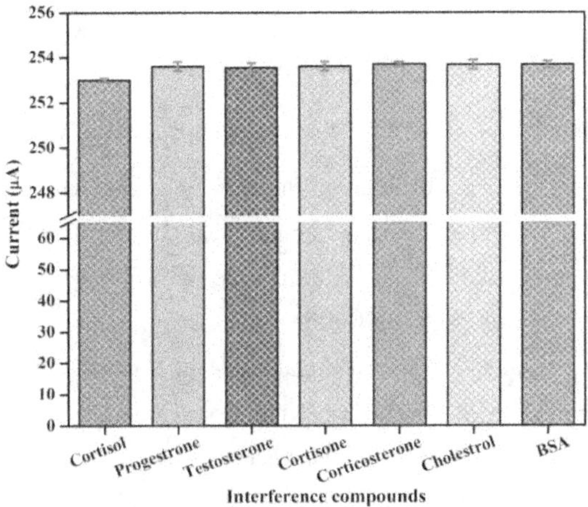

Fig. 3.14 Interference studies of BSA/Anti-C$_{mab}$/TiO$_2$/CCY immunoelectrode towards Progesterone, Testosterone, Cortisone, Corticosterone, Cholesterol and BSA towards cortisol (100 ng/mL) in PBS (10 mM, pH 7.0)

The selectivity of BSA/Anti-C_{mab}/TiO$_2$/CCY immunoelectrode with respect to interferents (100 ng/mL) such as progesterone, testosterone, corticosterone, cortisone, cholesterol and BSA with respect to cortisol (100 ng/mL) was studied using CV technique as shown in Fig. 3.14. TiO$_2$ nanocubes based immunosensor exhibited less cross-reactivity (± 3 μA) against each of the cortisol analogues including all other interference compounds.

3.4.7 Stability, repeatability and reproducibility studies

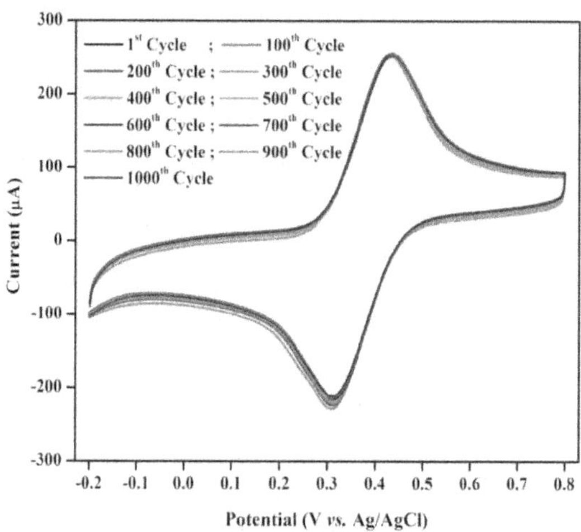

Fig. 3.15 The stability analysis of TiO$_2$/CCY immunoelectrode for 1000 cycles in 10 mM PBS

The accuracy and reproducibility of the immunosensor were also investigated by using CV technique. When not in use, the immunosensing electrodes were stored at 4 °C and examined for their electrochemical efficacy periodically by checking its relative activity. The results showed that there was no significance variation in its electrochemical activity over the period of 4 weeks, which retained 94.70 % of the initial current response. The RSD was calculated as 3.8 % from five repeated measurements with different BSA/Anti-C_{mab}/TiO$_2$/CCY immunosensor electrodes. The results ensured the reproducibility of the present method/immunosensor is quite suitable for clinical applications.

Also, the stability was investigated by measuring the electrochemical current response using CV for 1000 cycles in 10 mM PBS as shown in Fig. 3.15.

The corresponding RSD value was found less than 3.25 % for TiO_2/CCY immunoelectrode, which further proved the stability of the TiO_2/CCY fiber.

3.4.8 Real sample analysis

Table 3.1 Comparison of sweat cortisol estimated using chemiluminescence immunoassay and TiO_2/CCY based electrochemical immunosensor

Sweat Samples	CLIA method (ng/mL)	TiO₂/CCY immunosensor				
		Measured (ng/mL)*	Added (ng/mL)	Found (ng/mL)*	RSD (%)	Recovery (%)
1	46	41.56	50	95.78	5.836	104.60
2	34	36.42	50	84.85	4.673	98.18
3	58	56.12	50	101.89	3.064	96.01
4.	29	28.76	50	79.12	3.135	100.45
5.	24	30.94	50	82.86	3.346	102.37

*** The average value of three successive experiments.**

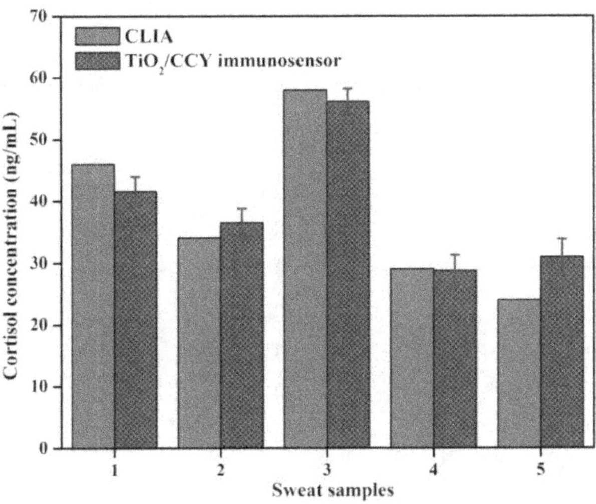

Fig. 3.16 Comparison graph of sweat cortisol estimated using chemiluminescence immunoassay and TiO_2/CCY based electrochemical immunosensor

The electrochemical response of BSA/Anti-C_{mab}/TiO$_2$/CCY immunosensor was further estimated the feasibility by measuring the recovery of spiked human sweat samples as given in Fig. 3.16. The outcomes were compared with the results obtained from commercially available CLIA method and summarized in Table 3.1. From the results, the RSD of the proposed immunosensor was determined for distinct real samples resulted in the range of 3.06-5.83% and the recovery rates of the samples was ranged between 96.01% and 104.60%. This result demonstrated that there was no significant variation observed between the proposed immunosensor and traditional CILA method.

3.5 Conclusions

In this chapter, we reported that the cortisol immunosensor made up of TiO$_2$ nanocubes and Anti-C_{mab}. TiO$_2$ nanocubes coated CCY provided larger surface area which facilitated more adsorption sites to Anti-C_{mab} for the effective interaction with the analyte compared to SnO$_2$ immunoelectrode due to its improved wettability. The prepared immunosensor showed good selectivity with minimal cross reactivity in presence of competing analogs molecules. Further, a satisfactory concurrence of analytical results of the designed BSA/Anti-C_{mab}/TiO$_2$/CCY immunosensor with those of standard CILA method showed good reliability. On the other hand, the value of surface area was measured lesser than that of SnO$_2$ which might be the reason for the electrochemical detection range and limit of the TiO$_2$/CCY based immunosensor could not offer higher sensitivity towards cortisol. This conclusion directed us to evaluate the catalytic performance of Fe$_2$O$_3$.

References

1. I. F. Akyildiz, W. Su, Y. Sankarasubramaniam, E. Cayirc, A survey on sensor networks, *IEEE Commun. Mag.,* **40** (2002) 102-104.

2. C. C. Shen, C. Srisathapornphat, C. Jaikaeo, Sensor Information Networking Architecture and Applications, *IEEE Pers. Commun.,* **8** (2001) 52–59.

3. P. S. Waggoner and H. G. Craighead, Micro and nanomechanical sensors for environmental, chemical and biological detection, *Lab Chip,* **7** (2007) 1238-1255.

4. D. Grieshaber, R. M. Kenzie, J. Vörös, E. Reimhult, Electrochemical biosensors - Sensor principles and architectures, *Sensors,* **8** (2008) 1400-1458.

5. J. Homola, Surface plasmon resonance sensors for detection of chemical and biological species, *Chem. Rev.,* **108** (2008) 462–493.

6. Z. R. Dai, Z. W. Pan, Z. L. Wang, Novel nanostructures of functional oxides synthesized by thermal evaporation, *Adv. Funct. Mater,* **13** (2003) 9-24.

7. N. Barsan, D. Koziej, U. Weimar, Metal oxide-based gas sensor research: How to?, *Sens. Actuator B-Chem.,* **121** (2007) 18-35.

8. D. A Tryk, A. Fujishima, K. Honda, Recent topics in photoelectrochemistry: achievements and future prospects, *Electrochim. Acta,* **45** (2000) 2363-2376.

9. A. Fujishima and K. Honda, Electrochemical photolysis of water at a semiconductor electrode, *Nature,* **238** (1972) 37–38.

10. A. Fujishima, T. N. Rao, D. A. Tryk, Titanium dioxide photocatalysis, *J. Photochem. Photobiol. C,* **1** (2000) 1-21.

11. J. Lin, Y. U. Heo, A. Nattesta, Z. Sun, L. Wang, J. H. Kim, S. X. Dou, 3D hierarchical rutile TiO_2 and metal-free organic sensitizer producing dye-sensitized solar cells 8.6% conversion efficiency, *Sci. Rep.,* **4** (2014) 5769.

12. X. Chen, L. Liu, Y. Y. Peter, S. S. Mao, Increasing solar absorption for photocatalysis with black hydrogenated titanium dioxide nanocrystals, *Science,* **331** (2011) 746–750.

13. I. Paramasivam, H. Jha, N. Liu, P. Schmuki, A review of photocatalysis using self-organized TiO_2 nanotubes and other ordered oxide nanostructures, *Small,* **8** (2012) 3073–3103.

14. M. H. Zarifi, S. Farsinezhad, M. Abdolrazzaghi, M. Daneshmand, K. Shankar, Selective microwave sensors exploiting the interaction of analytes with trap states in TiO_2 nanotube arrays, *Nanoscale,* **8** (2016) 7466–7473.

15. P. Si, S. Ding, J. Yuan, X. W. Lou, D. H. Kim, Hierarchically structured one-dimensional TiO_2 for protein immobilization, direct electrochemistry, and mediator-free glucose sensing, *ACS Nano,* **5** (2011) 7617–7626.

16. S. J. Bao, C. M. Li, J. F. Zang, X. Q. Cui, Y. Qiao, J. Guo, New nanostructured TiO_2 for direct electrochemistry and glucose sensor applications, *Adv. Funct. Mater.,* **18** (2008) 591–599.

17. A. Ghicova and P. Schmuki, Self-ordering electrochemistry: A review on growth and functionality of TiO_2 nanotubes and other self-aligned MOx structures, *Chem. Commun.,* **0** (2009) 2791-2808.

18. Y. Yin and A. P. Alivisatos, Colloidal nanocrystal synthesis and the organic-inorganic interface, *Nature,* **437** (2005) 664-670.

19. J. Bai and B. Zhou, Titanium dioxide nanomaterials for sensor applications, *Chem. Rev.,* **114** (2014) 10131−10176.

20. A. Norotsky, J. C. Jamieson, O. J. Kleppa, Enthalpy of transformation of a high pressure polymorph of titanium dioxide to the rutile modification, *Science,* **158** (1967) 338–389.

21. A. L. Linsebigler, G. Lu, J. T. Yates, Photocatalysis on TiO_2 surfaces: Principles, mechanisms, and selected results, *Chem. Rev.,* **95** (1995) 735–758.

22. W. Wunderlich, T. Oekermann, L. Miao, N. T. Hue, S. Tanemura, M. Tanemura, Electronic properties of Nano-porous TiO_2 and ZnO thin films comparison of simulations and experiments, *J. Ceram. Proc. Res.,* **5** (2004) 343–354.

23. A. Sclafani, L. Palmisano, M. Schiavello, Influence of the preparation methods of titanium dioxide on the photocatalytic degradation of phenol in aqueous dispersion, *J. Phys. Chem.,* **94** (1990) 829–832.

24. Q. Zhang, L. Gao and J. Guo, Effects of calcination on the photocatalytic properties of nanosized TiO_2 powders prepared by $TiCl_4$ hydrolysis, *Appl. Catal., B,* **26** (2000) 207-215.

25. S. Mo and W. Ching, Electronic and optical properties of three phases of titanium dioxide: Rutile, anatase and brookite, *Phys Rev B,* **51** (1995) 13023–13032.

26. J. Muscat, V. Swamy, N. M. Harrison, First-principles calculations of the phase stability of TiO_2, *Phy. Rev. B,* **65** (2002) 1–15.

27. Y. Hu, H.L Tsai, C.L Huang, Phase transformation of precipitated TiO_2 nanoparticles, *Mater. Sci. Eng. A,* **344** (2003) 209-214.

28. Y. Wang, T. Wu, Y. Zhou, C. Meng, W. Zhu, L. Liu, TiO_2 based nano heterostructures for promoting gas sensitivity performance: Designs, developments and prospects, *Sensors,* **17** (2017) 1971 (1-35).

29. S. Liu, Z. Wang, C. Yu, H. Bin, W. Gang, W. Q. Dong, J. Qiu, A. Eychmüller, X. W. Lou, A flexible $TiO_2(B)$-based battery electrode with superior power rate and ultralong cycle life, *Adv. Mater.,* **25** (2013) 3462-3467.

30. S. J. Bao, C. M. Li, J. F. Zang, X. Q. Cui, Y. Qiao, J. Guo, New nanostructured TiO_2 for direct electrochemistry and glucose sensor applications, *Adv Funct Mater.,* **18** (2008) 591-599.

31. J. Liu, Z. He, S. Y. Khoo, T. Thatt, Y. Tan, A new strategy for achieving vertically-erected and hierarchical TiO_2 nanosheets array/carbon cloth as a binder-free electrode for protein impregnation, direct electrochemistry and mediator-free glucose sensing, *Biosens. Bioelectron,* **77** (2016) 942–949.

32. P. Manickam, M. Sekar, R. Fernandez, C. Viswanathan, S. Bhansali, Fabric based wearable biosensor for continuous monitoring of steroids, *ECS Trans.,* **77** (2017) 1841-1846.

33. E. Hosono, S. Fujihara, K. Kakiuchi, H. Imai, Growth of submicrometer-scale rectangular parallelepiped rutile TiO_2 films in aqueous $TiCl_3$ solutions under hydrothermal conditions, *J. Am. Chem. Soc.,* **126** (2004) 7790–7791.

34. W. Guo, C. Xu, X. Wang, S. Wang, C. Pan, C. Lin, Z. L. Wang, Rectangular bunched rutile TiO$_2$ nanorod arrays grown on carbon fiber for dye-sensitized solar cells, *J. Am. Chem. Soc.*, **134** (2012) 4437–4441.

35. S. S. Mali, C. A. Betty, P. N. Bhosale, P. S. Patil, Hydrothermal synthesis of rutile TiO$_2$ with hierarchical microspheres and their characterization, *CrystEngComm.*, **13** (2011) 6349–6351.

36. L. Kavan, B. O' Regan, A. Kay, M. Grätzel, Preparation of TiO$_2$ (anatase) films on electrodes by anodic oxidative hydrolysis of TiCl$_3$, *J. Electroanal. Chem.*, **346** (1993) 291-307.

37. S. S. Mali, H. Kim, C. S. Shim, P. S. Patil, J. H. Kim, C. K. Hong, Surfactant free most probable TiO$_2$ nanostructures via hydrothermal and its dye sensitized solar cell properties, *Sci. Rep.*, **3** (2004), 1-8.

38. X. Wu, Z. Chen, G. Q. Lu and L. Wang, Solar cells: nanosized anatase TiO$_2$ single crystals with tunable exposed (001) facets for enhanced energy conversion efficiency of dye-Sensitized Solar Cells, *Adv. Funct. Mater.*, **21** (2011) 4166–4166.

39. M. H. Jung, M. J. Chu and M. G. Kang, TiO$_2$ nanotube fabrication with highly exposed (001) facets for enhanced conversion efficiency of solar cells, *Chem. Commun.*, **48** (2012) 5016–5018.

40. Q. Huang and L. Gao, A simple route for the synthesis of rutile TiO$_2$ nanorods, *Chem. Lett.*, **32** (2003) 638-639.

41. S. Liu, Z. Luo, G. Tian, M. Zhu , Z. Cai , A. Pan , S. Liang, TiO$_2$ nanorods grown on carbon fiber cloth as binder-free electrode for sodium-ion batteries and flexible sodium-ion capacitors, *J. Power Sources*, **363** (2017) 284-290.

42. L. Yang, Z. Hong, J. Wu, L. W. Zhu, Facile production of a large-area flexible TiO$_2$/carbon cloth for dye removal, *RSC Adv.*, **4** (2014) 25556–25561.

43. H. Meng, W. Hou, X. Xu, J. Xu, X. Zhang, TiO$_2$-loaded activated carbon fiber: Hydrothermal synthesis, adsorption properties and photo catalytic activity under visible light irradiation, *Particuology*, **14** (2014) 38–43

44. S. Madhu, P. Manickam, M. Pierre, S. Bhansali, P. Nagamony, V. Chinnuswamy, Nanostructured SnO_2 integrated conductive fabrics as binder-free electrode for neurotransmitter detection, *Sens. Actuators A,* **269** (2018) 401–411.

45. B. Xing, C. Shi, C. Zhang, G. Yi, L. Chen, H. Guo, G. Huang, J. Cao, Preparation of TiO_2/Activated carbon composites for photocatalytic degradation of RhB under UV Light irradiation, *J Nanomater.,* **8393648** (2016) 1-10.

46. Y. Yang, M. Qiu, L. Liu, TiO_2 nanorod array@carbon cloth photocatalyst for CO_2 reduction, *Ceram. Int.,* **42** (2016) 15081–15086.

47. R.J. Meier, Vibrational spectroscopy: a "vanishing" discipline?, *Chem. Soc. Rev.,* **34** (2005) 743–752.

48. S. K. Arya, A. Dey, S. Bhansali, Polyaniline protected gold nanoparticles-based mediator and label free electrochemical cortisol biosensor, *Biosens. Bioelectron,* **28** (2011) 166–173.

Chapter IV

Ellipsoidal Fe₂O₃ Integrated Carbon Fiber Based Electrochemical Immunosensor for Ultrasensitive Sweat Cortisol Measurement

Highlights

- Fe_2O_3 nanostructures were integrated with flexible carbon yarn by simple hydrothermal method.

- Fe_2O_3/CCY flexible and binder free electrode has been used for electrochemical cortisol estimation.

- The obtained working range and detection limit are 1 fg - 1 μg and 0.005 fg, respectively.

- The practical applicability of Fe_2O_3/CCY also assured the effective non-invasive quantification of cortisol in human sweat.

Graphical illustration of immobilization and electrochemical immunosensing of cortisol on hydrothermally derived Fe₂O₃ /CCY with possible redox mechanism

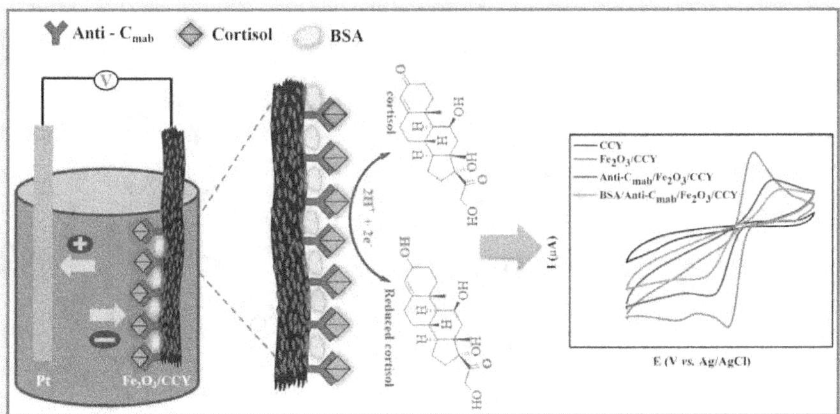

4.1 Introduction

Nanostructured magnetic materials with preferred size and shape play a vital role in modern science and technology [1]. Amongst the various nanostructured materials, highly crystalline magnetic nanostructures with various sizes and morphologies are attracting considerable attention due to their low effective density, high specific surface area, intriguing size- and shape-dependent properties, superior permeation and attractive potential applications in the fields of magnetics, catalysis, water treatment, energy storage, drug delivery and distinct sensor applications [2-7].

Hematite (α-Fe_2O_3) is one of the semiconducting magnetic nanomaterials which is most stable under ambient conditions with n-type semiconducting properties. It has been investigated extensively above said wide range of applications due to its abundance, low cost, high stability and environmental benignity with great scientific and technical features [8-10]. Inspired by its outstanding characteristics, much effort has been made to prepare the nanostructured α-Fe_2O_3 with different sizes and shapes because of its strong size and shape dependent properties. In this direction, various well-defined α-Fe_2O_3 nanostructures with different dimensionalities such as nanoparticles, nano and microspheres, nanocubes, nanotubes, nanorods, hollow nanostructures and nanoplates have been accomplished [11-15].

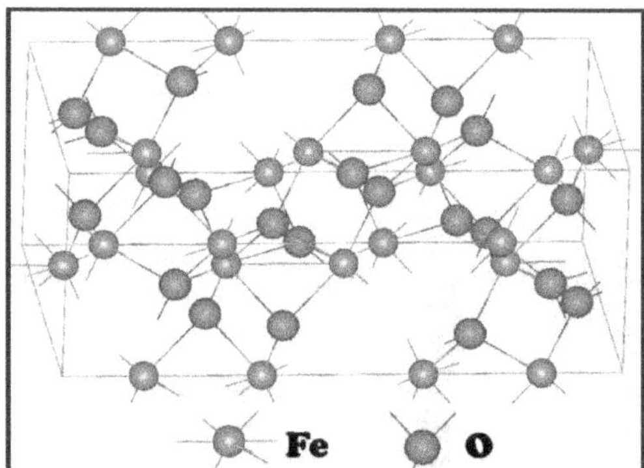

Fig. 4.1 Crystal structure of α-Fe_2O_3

The controlled synthesis of uniform α-Fe_2O_3 nanostructures has fascinated considerable interest and many methods have been developed [16, 17]. Sol-gel process, gas-solid growth route, hydrothermal approach, chemical precipitation, high energy ball milling, thermal oxidation at high temperature and microwave heat method are employed widely to prepare the α-Fe$_2$O$_3$ nanostructures with various shapes and sizes [18-24].

Hydrothermal synthesis is an attractive technique among these methods with several advantages: (i) effective control of size, morphology and degree of agglomeration of the particles, (ii) relatively low reaction temperature (iii) materials with high purity incorporation (iv) an environmentally benign route and (v) a cost-effective [25].

X. Wang *et al.,* developed a facile and scalable strategy to prepare core-shell Fe$_2$O$_3$/carbon cloth (CC) structure using hydrothermal route and used it as binder free electrode for LIBs. The developed hierarchical porous Fe$_2$O$_3$ nanorods on the CC can effectively shorten the transfer paths of lithium ions and reduced the contact resistance. Promoted from the particular electrode architecture, Fe$_2$O$_3$@C/CC as anode without the use of polymer any binder and conductive agent exhibited excellent electrochemical performances [26]. L. Ji *et al.,* have demonstrated highly dispersed α-Fe$_2$O$_3$ nanoparticles with an average size of 20 nm were successfully loaded in carbon nanofibers through cost effective electro-spinning and thermal treatment processes and the same as used binder-free anode materials for rechargeable LIBs. The developed nano phases exhibited a high reversible capacity of about 604 mAh g^{-1} at 50 mAg^{-1}, improved capacity retention for at least 100 cycles and enhanced rate performance even at the high current density of 500 mA g^{-1} [27]. Recently, K. P. O. Mahesh *et al.,* (2018) reported that the porous Fe$_2$O$_3$ nanoparticles are directly grown on CC using a simple hydrothermal method for employment as a flexible and wearable electrochemical electrode for the detection of dopamine. They achieved of an impressively low LOD of 50 nM for DA and concluded Fe$_2$O$_3$ deposited flexible CC electrode is a promising candidate for designing inexpensive wearable biosensors for the detection of other analytes [28].

Therefore, a novel design of the structure with Fe$_2$O$_3$ nanostructure coated on flexible CCY flexible substrate is highly desirable to achieve the binder free electrode with high electrochemical sensing performance. With these motivations in this *chapter IV*, we have prepared ellipsoidal α-Fe$_2$O$_3$ nanostructures on flexible CCY platform for developing electrochemical immunosensors to monitor cortisol levels. Anti-C$_{mab}$ were immobilized onto the Fe$_2$O$_3$/CCY electrode using EDC/NHS chemistry. The fabricated immunosensor was tested for cortisol level in human sweat samples and validated with commercial CLIA method.

4.2 Materials and methods

4.2.1 Chemicals and reagents

Iron (III) chloride Hexahydrate (FeCl$_3$.6H$_2$O), Pluronic f127 (PEO$_{100}$PPO$_{70}$PEO$_{100}$) were purchased from sigma Aldirch. All the chemicals were of analytical grade and were used without further purification.

Bleached and scoured CCY with the density of 0.35 g/cm^3 and diameter of ~350 µm was purchased from Vinpro Tech, Hyderabad, India. The purchased CCY was ultrasonicated and dried at ambient temperature under vacuum for 24 hrs to remove any impurities prior to characterization and material deposition.

4.2.2 Synthesis of ellipsoidal Fe$_2$O$_3$ nanostructures integration on CCY (Fe$_2$O$_3$/CCY)

Ellipsoidal Fe$_2$O$_3$ was integrated on CCY using the effective hydrothermal method, wherein stoichiometric amounts of pluronic f127 were added to an aqueous solution of FeCl$_3$.6H$_2$O under continuing magnetic stirring. Following this, the obtained homogeneous solution was transferred into a Teflon vial (65 mL). CCY was immersed in this solution and placed in a sealed autoclave followed by 12 hrs heat treatment at 180 °C. The resulting yarn was allowed to cool down to room temperature naturally and washed with alcohol, double distilled water for four times to remove remaining impurities. Then the product was dried at 60 °C overnight and the entire process has been illustrated in scheme 1.

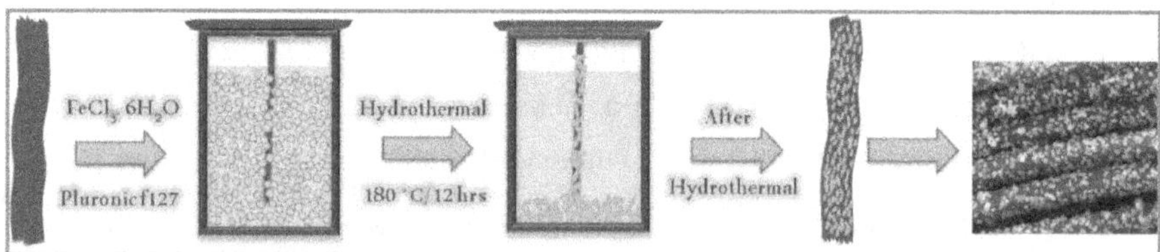

Scheme 1 Schematic illustration of synthesis of Fe$_2$O$_3$ on CCY by hydrothermal method

4.2.3 Immobilization of Anti-C$_{mab}$ onto Fe$_2$O$_3$/CCY electrode

A standard process reported previously has been utilized to immobilize Anti-C$_{mab}$ covalently onto Fe$_2$O$_3$/CCY electrode [29]. The immobilization of Anti-C$_{mab}$ with

Fe_2O_3/CCY electrode was achieved via electrostatic interaction using EDC as the coupling agent and NHS as the activator. To fabricate the electrochemical immunosensor electrode, 70 µL of 2 µg/mL, Anti-C_{mab} solution was mixed with the Fe_2O_3/CCY in 5 mL PBS (10 mM, pH 7.0) solution containing 0.4 M NHS and 0.4 M EDC and incubated for 120 mins in a humid chamber. The fabricated Anti-C_{mab}/Fe_2O_3/CCY electrode was washed with PBS (10 mM, pH 7.0) to remove the loosely bound molecules. Following this the sensor electrode was immersed in 50 µL of BSA (10 µg/mL) in PBS (10 mM, pH 7.0) and incubated for 30 mins for blocking the non bound sites on the Anti-C_{mab}/Fe_2O_3/CCY electrode surface. As fabricated BSA/Anti-C_{mab}/Fe_2O_3/CCY immunoelectrode was further washed using PBS (10 mM, pH 7.0) and stored at 4 °C.

4.2.4 Growth mechanism of α-Fe_2O_3 on CCY

Pluronic F127 is one of these types of triblock copolymers consisting of the two monomers in the arrangement $PEO_{100}PPO_{65}PEO_{100}$. The possible growth mechanism of ellipsoidal Fe_2O_3 nanostructures on CCY was given in scheme 2.

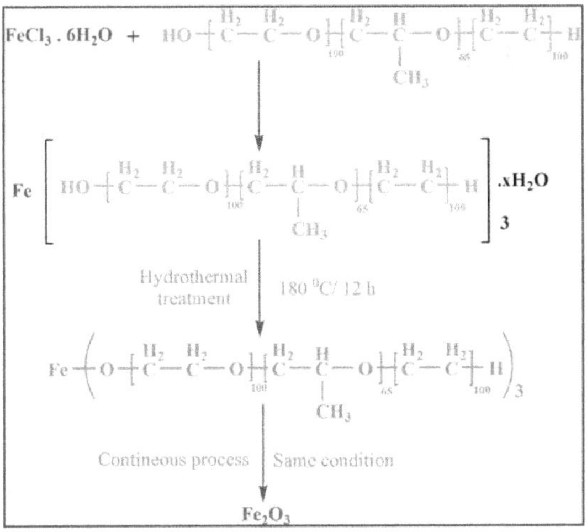

Scheme 2. Possible formation mechanism of α-Fe_2O_3 on CCY by hydrothermal method

It has been reported that alkylene oxide segments in the Pluronic triblock copolymer are capable of forming crown ether-type complexes with metal ions, resulting in coordination bonds between copolymer and inorganic nanoparticles. Thus, in our route Pluronic 127 is designed as the assembling reagent via the coordination bonding with hematite (α-Fe_2O_3) nanoparticles [30].

4.3 Results and Discussion

4.3.1 XRD analysis of CCY and Fe_2O_3/CCY

The crystal structure and phases of the prepared samples were investigated by XRD measurements and the resulting diffraction patterns are displayed in Fig. 4.2. The bare CCY showed only two broad diffraction peaks at 25.8° and 43.6° which could be indexed to the (002) and (100) planes of amorphous carbon, respectively [31, 32]. For Fe_2O_3/CCY, the signature patterns for carbon yarn was observed at 25.9° (002) along with other diffraction peaks at 24.2°, 33.2° (major), 35.86°, 40.96° and 54.13° corresponding to (012), (104), (110), (113) and (116) planes of Fe_2O_3, respectively. The result was consistent with the standard XRD pattern of rhombohedral α-Fe_2O_3 (JCPDS No. 84-0309) which proved that the successful formation of Fe_2O_3 on CCY with high purity [33]. The average grain size of Fe_2O_3 on CCY is $\sim$ 12 nm which was calculated using Scherrer's formula (Eq. 2.4) according to the diffraction peak of Fe_2O_3 (104) plane.

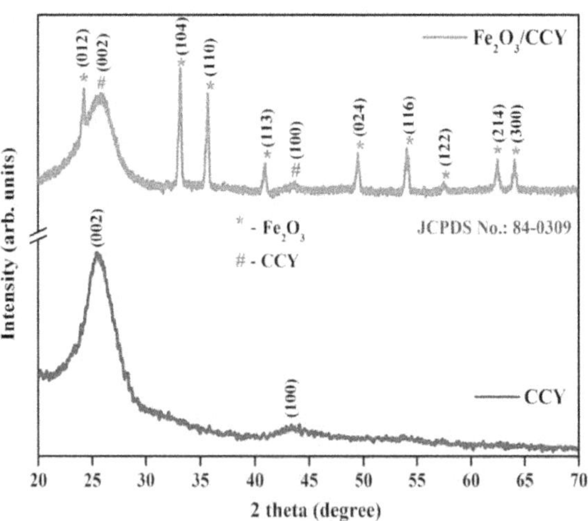

Fig. 4.2 X-ray diffraction patterns of CCY and α-Fe_2O_3/CCY

4.3.2 FT-IR spectra of CCY and α-Fe₂O₃/CCY

In order to investigate the interaction between Fe₂O₃ and CCY, the FT-IR spectra have been taken. For pristine CCY, a characteristic peak at 1585 cm⁻¹ was attributed from C=C stretching and the band appeared around 1063 cm⁻¹ was related to C–C stretching vibration in the carbon. The peaks at 787 cm⁻¹, 2851 and 2912 cm⁻¹ were ascribed to the bending and stretching vibrations of the C-H bond. A strong absorption band at 3410 cm⁻¹ corresponds to O-H stretching vibration of surface adsorbed water molecule along with residual O-H bending at 1390 cm⁻¹ respectively [34]. The peak at and deformation vibration at 1730 cm⁻¹ corresponding to presence of C=O in CCY [35, 36]. The absorption band at 574 cm⁻¹ is attributed to the Fe-OH bond vibration, present in Fe₂O₃ integrated CCY. In addition, weak peak around 1413 cm⁻¹ roots in C-O deformation vibration, implying the existence of intramolecular hydrogen bonding between CCY and Fe-OH, which is beneficial in keeping the stability of material structure. A remarkable decrement in the absorption of C=O, O-H (deformation vibration) and the C-O groups were observed, proving that most of the oxygen containing groups were removed in Fe₂O₃/CCY [37]. From the FT-IR results, we corroborate that the Fe₂O₃ are covered to the CCY surface uniformly.

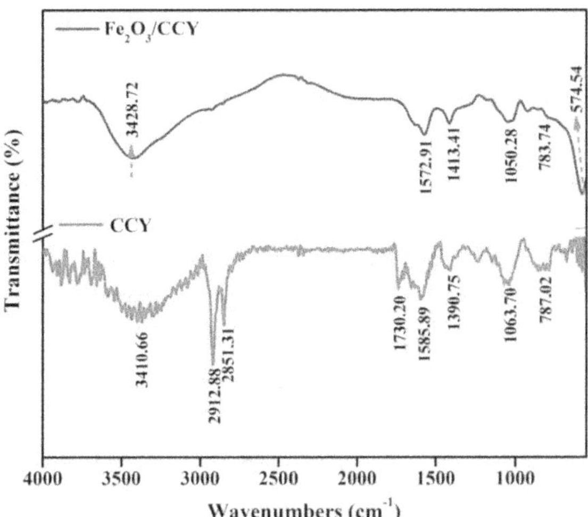

Fig. 4.3 FT-IR spectra of CCY and Fe₂O₃/CCY

4.3.3 RAMAN spectra of CCY and Fe$_2$O$_3$/CCY

Raman spectroscopy was used to further confirm the structural characteristics of prepared electrode materials and the results are shown in Fig. 4.4. The D-band located at 1354 cm^{-1} and the G-band at 1594 cm^{-1} are the characteristic Raman peaks of carbon, which can be observed in both pure CCY and Fe$_2$O$_3$/CCY. The G band assigned to the first order scattering of the E$_{2g}$ phonon of CCY represent the in plane bond stretching vibration of sp^2 bonded carbon atoms in a 2D hexagonal lattice. The D band is associated with the breathing mode of K-point phonons of A$_{1g}$ symmetry with vibration of carbon atoms with angling bonds in plane terminations of disordered carbon yarn [38]. As we can see from the spectra of Fe$_2$O$_3$/CCY, the Fe$_2$O$_3$ sample exhibited the bands at 230, 296, 410 and 610 cm^{-1} indicating the presence of Fe$_2$O$_3$ (hematite) phase with the D$^6{}_{3d}$ crystal space group [39, 40]. These results implied a tight integration of Fe$_2$O$_3$ nanostructures on CCY and supporting the XRD results very well.

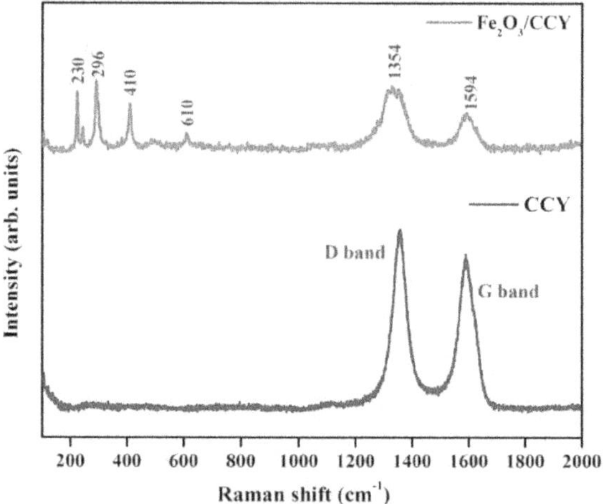

Fig. 4.4 Raman spectra of CCY and Fe$_2$O$_3$/CCY

4.3.4 Morphological and compositional analysis of CCY and Fe$_2$O$_3$/CCY

The morphology of the CCY and Fe$_2$O$_3$/CCY were elucidated by FESEM analysis and the corresponding images are shown in Fig. 4.5. As seen in Fig. 4.5(a), the morphology of pure CCY is consists of smaller fibers and revealed that there was no impurity on the smooth surface. The inset shows the clearer version of the smooth fiber. The high magnification of FESEM images shown in Fig. 4.5(b–d) provide clear information about the ellipsoidal Fe_2O_3 nanostructures.

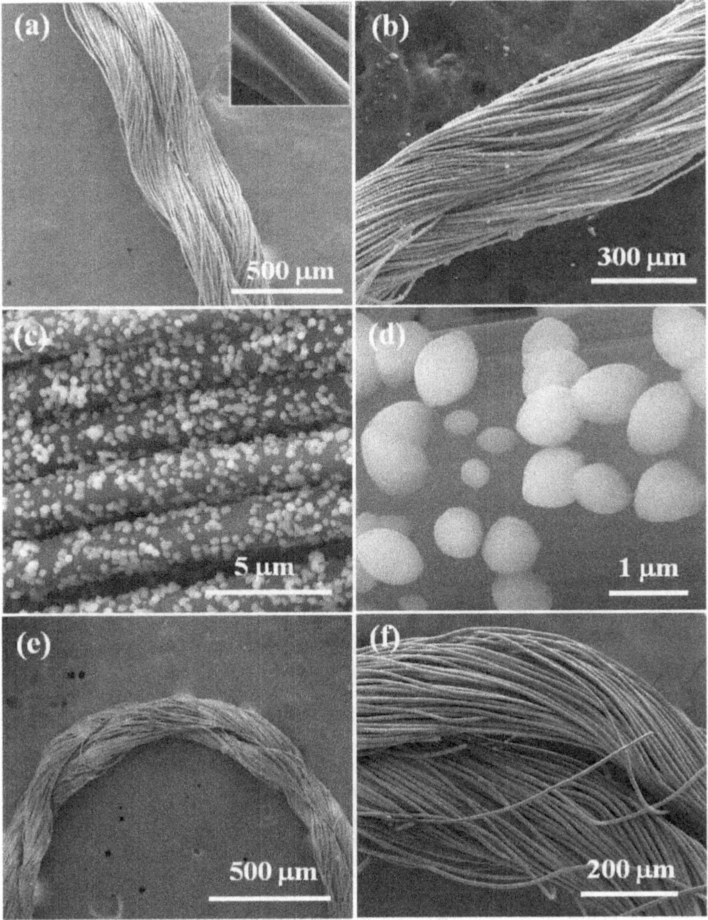

Fig. 4.5 FESEM images of (a) bare CCY, (b-d) Fe_2O_3/CCY and (e&f) Fe_2O_3/CCY electrode freely rolled up with tweezers

As depicted the carbon yarn surfaces are uniformly covered by uniform sized Fe_2O_3 ellipsoids with the diameter of 300-350 nm and the length of ~ 800-850 nm. The large number of Fe_2O_3 nanoparticles were uniformly anchored onto the carbon yarn surface via self-assembly due to the differences in surface charges resulting in strong electrostatic interactions, which is expected to improve the electrochemical properties of Fe_2O_3 resulting in enhanced sensing performance.

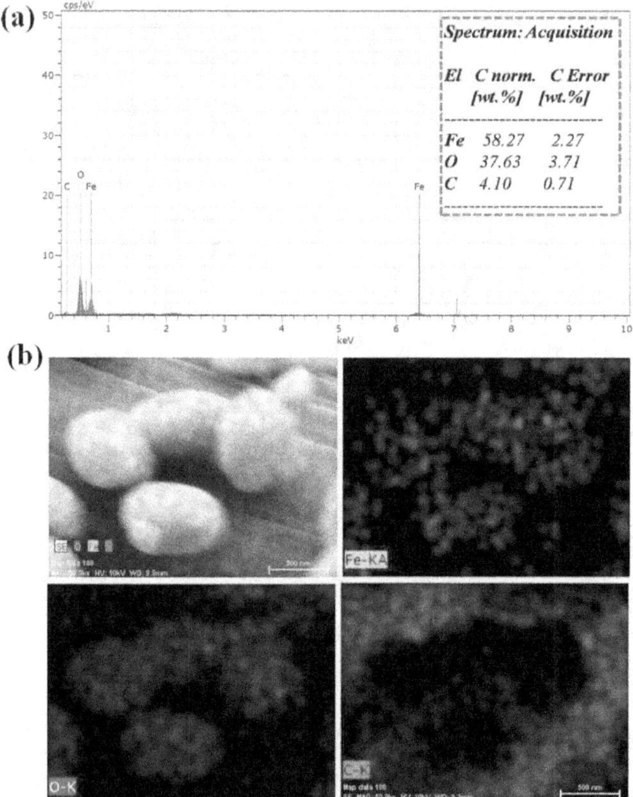

Fig. 4.6 (a) EDS spectra and (b) EDS mapping of Fe_2O_3/CCY

Moreover, the presence of void spaces between adjacent nano-ellipsoids would facilitate the electrolyte diffusion and enhance the electro-active sites. It is illustrated that interfacial interaction between the carbon fiber substrate and Fe_2O_3 nanoellipsoid is so strong that the Fe_2O_3 nanoellipsoid are not easily detached from carbon fibers even after ultrasonication for 5 min [41].

Thereby, the oxygen functional groups and rich defective sites existing on the carbon fibers by hydrothermal treatment are particularly favorable for the initial nucleation of FeOOH at defective sites, most important to homogeneous distribution of C, O and Fe elements in the whole CCY surface [42]. Fig. 4.5 (e and f) showed images of the integrated ellipsoidal Fe_2O_3/CCY electrode which can be freely rolled up with tweezers. It can be clearly observed that the electrodes exhibit excellent flexibility, which makes them to be used in flexible and wearable devices. The successful synthesis of Fe_2O_3 ellipsoid on CCY and its chemical composition was further confirmed from EDS mapping analysis. As shown in Fig. 4.6a, Fe and O are the two elements coated on CCY apart from the carbon that relates to the substrate. Moreover, elemental mapping technique shown in Fig. 4.6b further established the homogeneous coating of the yarn with Fe_2O_3 nanoparticles.

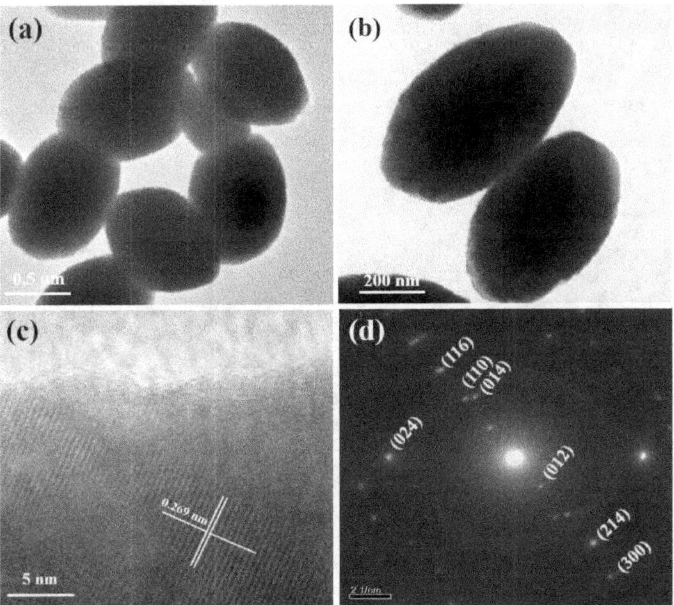

Fig. 4.7 HRTEM images (a-c) and SAED pattern (d) of Fe_2O_3 nanoparticles

To extensively study the morphology of the Fe_2O_3 nanostructures, we have used the HRTEM imaging and selected area electron diffraction (SAED) analysis. Figure 4.7 (a & b) depicts the typical HRTEM images of Fe_2O_3 nanoparticles and indicated the ellipsoidal morphology with a homogeneously well dispersed structure which is consistent with the FESEM micrograph. The ellipsoidal Fe_2O_3 nanostructure was beneficial for electrode materials due to the large surface area. In Fig. 4.7c the uniform lattice structure without detectable defects and the calculated d spacing of 0.269 nm corresponds to the (104) planes of hematite could be clearly observed which can be correlated with XRD data. The corresponding SAED pattern is shown in Fig. 4.7d which indicated the polycrystalline nature of Fe_2O_3.

4.3.5 Electrical and mechanical properties of CCY and Fe_2O_3/CCY

The electrical resistance of 5 cm long CCY and Fe_2O_3 coated CCY were measured to examine their electrical properties. The resistance of the Fe_2O_3/CCY (58±1.2 Ω) increased when compared to the untreated CCY (36 ±1 Ω). The conductivity of Fe_2O_3/CCY was demonstrated by powering an LED device connected to a battery as shown in Fig. 4.8. The average weight of Fe_2O_3 was measured by checking the weight of CCY before and after Fe_2O_3 hydrothermal deposition and the weight of 5 cm length CCY and Fe_2O_3/CCY are 1.23 and 2.1 mg respectively.

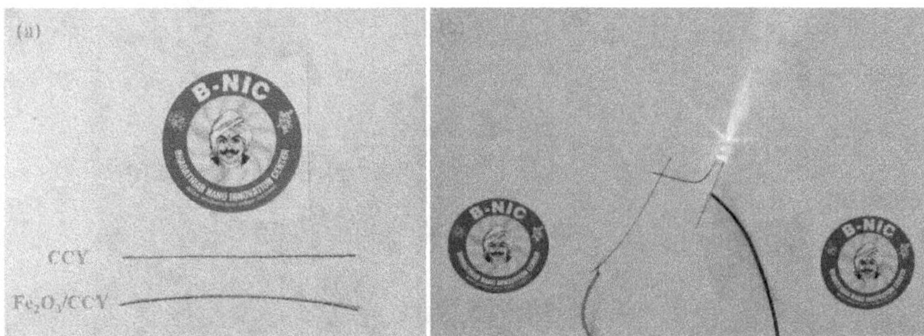

Fig. 4.8 Photographs of CCY– Fe_2O_3/CCY; (a) Comparison of the pure CCY and Fe_2O_3 Coated CCY (b) Demonstration of LED emission with the current passing through Fe_2O_3 coated yarn

The mechanical properties of CCY and Fe_2O_3/CCY electrodes were investigated for its tensile, elongation and elastic modulus properties. The ultimate strength measured for Fe_2O_3/CCY is found to be 33.27 MPa and this value is higher than of pristine CCY (20.10 MPa). This indicates that the strength of the fiber is improved when it is modified with Fe_2O_3. Similarly, elongation and young's modulus of the Fe_2O_3/CCY was 20.40 % and 67.03 MPa were improved after Fe_2O_3 inclusion (7.53 % and 37.17 MPa). It further confirmed the flexibility of the modified fibers.

4.3.6 Specific and assessable surface area of CCY and α-Fe_2O_3/CCY electrode

The BET surface area of the CCY and Fe_2O_3/CCY found to be 75.607 m^2/g and 146.02 m^2/g respectively. The uniform Fe_2O_3 nano-ellipsoids on CCY exhibited two fold increased the surface area compared to bare CCY. The high specific surface area of Fe_2O_3/CCY was calculated using BET analysis which is higher than the other morphologies given in the previous reports.

The electrochemically accessible active surface area (A_e) of CCY and Fe_2O_3/CCY were calculated using the standard Randle–Sevcik equation (Eq. 2.3). The calculated A_e values (bare CCY is 0.0700 cm^2 and Fe_2O_3/CCY is 0.0942 cm^2) also ensured the high sensitivity of the prepared electrode. Thus, the higher surface area of Fe_2O_3 on CCY may play a vital role in their electrochemical performance.

4.3.7 Wettability analysis of CCY and Fe_2O_3/CCY

Moreover, applicability of the prepared α-Fe_2O_3/CCY in wearable sensor applications, its surface feature was analyzed using contact angle measurement. We have characterized the wettability of CCY and Fe_2O_3 coated CCY by acquiring images of sessile water drops cast on the Fe_2O_3 coated CCY by a custom setup with a charge-coupled device (CCD) camera. Static advanced contact angles were measured the volume of the drop by a 2 μL. As shown in Fig. 4.9 the contact angles of water on bare CCY was obtained 151.0° ±1.1, suggesting a highly hydrophobic surface nature of CCY. In contrast, water can rapidly spread over the Fe_2O_3 coated CCY substrate once it contact with the substrate which implied an improved wetting ability after hydrothermal treatment; then observed contact angle was nearly 0° (Fig. 4.9).

In nature, water droplets on a lotus leaf tend to remain balanced on the top of micro-/nanosized surface structures, due to entrapped air pockets; this is referred to as the Fakir state [43]. However, if Fe_2O_3 nanoellipsoid could be wetted well by a polar solution, such as water, there would be used in the area of biosensor and supercapacitor electrodes because of its enlarged wetted area in a buffer solution [44].

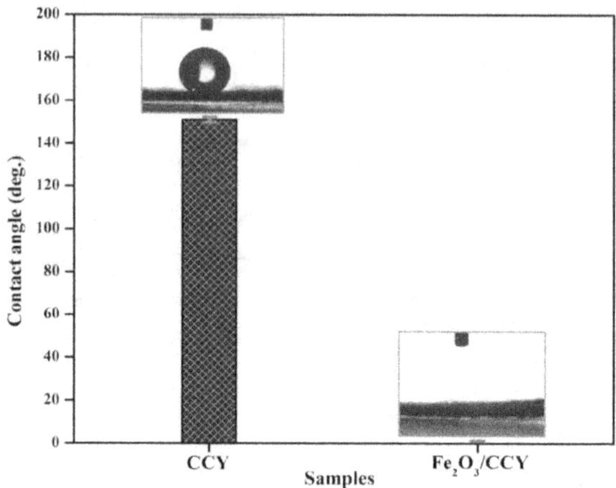

Fig. 4.9 Water contact angle on CCY and Fe_2O_3 modified CCY [Insets: The images of water droplet with contact angle]

4.3.8 *In vitro* cell viability evaluation

Fibroblasts are widely distributed in many types of tissues, such as tendon, ligament and skin. Fibroblasts are traditionally defined as the cells that produce collagens and are considered to be the primary source of most extracellular matrix components. They play a critical role in regulating the turnover of extracellular matrix and play an important part in wound healing. Fibroblasts are able to differentiate to myofibroblasts, specialized cells that possess a contractile phenotype with α-smooth muscle action expression. Myofibroblasts are responsible for the generation of the contraction forces that allow wound contraction during wound healing process

For the wearable sensor applications, the Fe_2O_3 coated CCY have been widely documented with different concentrations of 0.25, 0.5 and 1 mg for cytotoxicity analysis. Fig. 4.10 shows the *in vitro* fibroblast L929 cell viability cultured with the pristine CCY and Fe_2O_3 coated CCY in DMSO. After 24 hrs incubation, it was found that Fe_2O_3/CCY did not negatively influences the cell viability even at higher concentrations, which suggested that Fe_2O_3 deposited CCY have reasonably good biocompatibility to mouse fibroblast L929 cells. These data ensured the non-toxic property of prepared Fe_2O_3/CCY, thus it could be used as an excellent sensor platform in smart textiles.

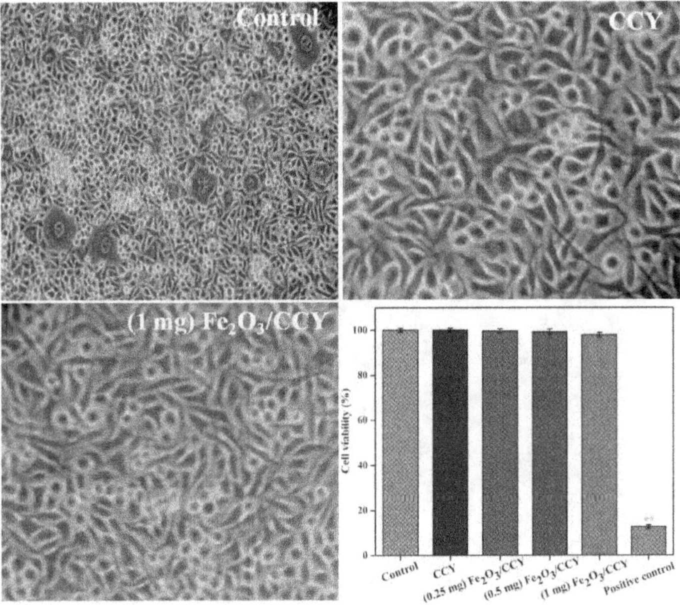

Fig. 4.10 MTT analysis of cultured fibroblast L929 cells treated with different concentration of Fe_2O_3 nanoellipsoid on CCY samples for 24 hrs. Data represented as mean ± SD of three independent tests. **$P<0.01$

4.4 Electrochemical analysis

4.4.1 Cyclic voltammetry studies

The obtained Fe_2O_3/CCY was directly applied as a working electrode to evaluate its electrochemical cortisol sensing performance. CV study was used to examine the electro activity of the functionalized electrode to understand the electrochemical behavior of the electrode. Fig. 4.11 shows the CV studies of the bare CCY, Fe_2O_3/CCY, Anti-C_{mab}/Fe_2O_3/CCY and BSA/Anti-C_{mab}/Fe_2O_3/CCY immuneolectrode in PBS (10 mM, pH 7.0). The bare CCY exhibited oxidation and reduction current magnitude in the range of $\sim 10^{-6}$ A, which is a typical characteristic of bare CCY. The redox current response increased to ~292.7 µA for Fe_2O_3/CCY electrode and the anodic peak corresponds to the oxidation of Fe^{2+} to Fe^{3+} and the cathodic peak corresponds to the reduction of Fe^{3+} to Fe^{2+}.

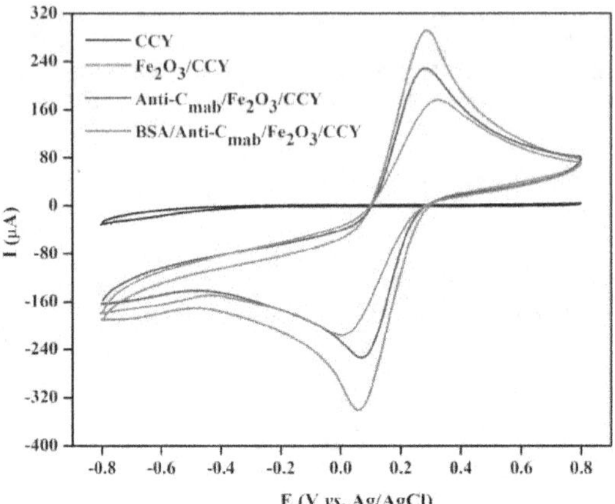

Fig. 4.11 CV analysis of step wise fabrication of BSA/Anti-C$_{mab}$/ Fe$_2$O$_3$/CCY immunoelectrode from CCY in PBS (10 mM, pH 7.0)

The magnitude of current response decreased to ~228.99 µA after the immobilization of Anti-C$_{mab}$ onto Fe$_2$O$_3$/CCY electrode confirmed the binding of Anti-C$_{mab}$. The decreased current response was due to the hindrance of electron charge caused by the insulating nature of antibodies. Moreover, the electrochemical oxidation peak current response of BSA/Anti-C$_{mab}$/Fe$_2$O$_3$/CCY immunoelectrode was observed to be lower than that of Anti-C$_{mab}$/Fe$_2$O$_3$/CCY immunoelectrode. The BSA also was used to block the non-binding sites and thereby provided selective interaction of Anti-C$_{mab}$/Fe$_2$O$_3$/CCY immunoelectrode with the analyte.

4.4.2 Effect of pH

To investigate the optimal pH, the activity of BSA/Anti-C$_{mab}$/Fe$_2$O$_3$/CCY immunoelectrode was investigated in the pH range of 6.0 to 8.0 in PBS (Fig. 4.12a). It was observed that the oxidation and reduction peak current decreased while increasing the pH from 6.0 - 7.0. Beyond the pH 7.0, the peak current again linearly increased (as shown in Fig. 4.12b) upto pH 8.0. However, it was observed the most stable oxidation and reduction peak area and current response was high for pH 7.0. Thus, pH 7.0 was selected as the working electrolyte pH, which mimics biological conditions. It has been chosen as the optimal pH for following successive experiments.

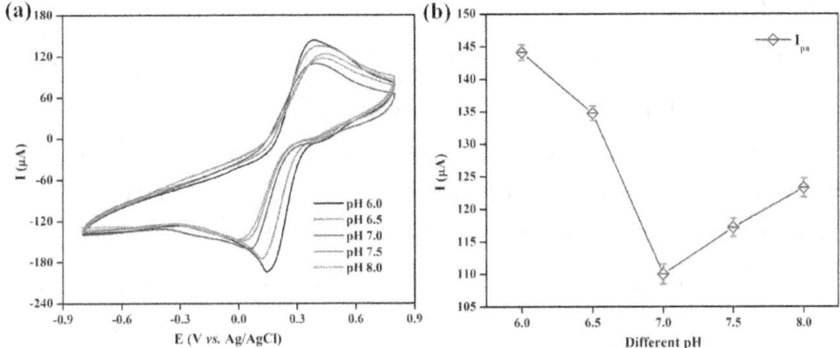

Fig. 4.12 (a) CV analysis of the BSA/Anti-C$_{mab}$/ Fe$_2$O$_3$/CCY immunoelectrode as a function of pH from 4.5 to 8.5 in PBS and (b) Linear plots of peak current *vs.* pH values

4.4.3 Effect of scan rate

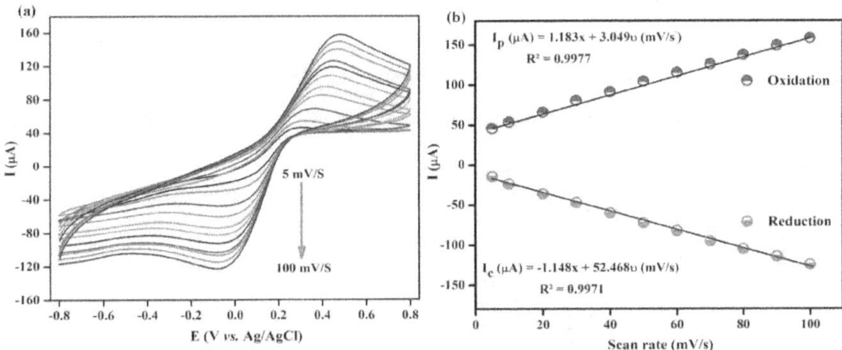

Fig. 4.13 (a) CV analysis of the BSA/Anti-C$_{mab}$/Fe$_2$O$_3$/CCY immunoelectrode as a function of scan rates (5 to 100 mV/s) in PBS (10 mM, pH 7.0) and (b) Linear plot of the oxidation and reduction peak currents *vs.* square root of scan rates

The electrochemical behavior of the BSA/Anti-C$_{mab}$/Fe$_2$O$_3$/CCY immunoelectrode was also studied using CV as a function of scan rates from 5-100 mV/s in PBS (10 mM, pH 7.0) which is shown in Fig. 4.13a and the change in anodic and cathodic current response with scan rate was plotted in Fig. 4.13b. It is observed that the magnitude of the current was linearly varied with the scan rates and the corresponding equations are given in Eq. 4.1 & 4.2.

$$I_{pa} \ (\mu A) = 1.183x + 3.049\upsilon \ (mV \ s^{-1}); \quad R^2 = 0.9977 \quad ---- \ (Eq. \ 4.1)$$

$$I_{pc} \ (\mu A) = -1.148x + 52.468\upsilon \ (mV \ s^{-1}); \ R^2 = 0.9971 \quad ---- \ (Eq. \ 4.2)$$

The well-defined redox peak suggested that the diffusion of electron was surface controlled. The separation of peaks suggested that the process was not perfectly reversible but the stable redox peak current and position during the repeated scans at a particular scan rate implied that the immunoelectrode displayed a quasi-reversible process [45].

The obtained low working potential could also help to avoid possible interference from the biological samples. It was found that at a scan rate of 50 mV/s, the electrode exhibited stability and equal oxidation and reduction peak area and current values. Thus, all further CV studies were carried out at a scan rate of 50 mV/s.

4.4.4 Cortisol response studies of BSA/Anti-C$_{mab}$/Fe$_2$O$_3$/CCY immunoelectrode by CV

The electrochemical response of BSA/Anti-C$_{mab}$/Fe$_2$O$_3$/CCY immunoelectrode has been studied using CV technique using PBS (pH 7.0, 10 mM) as a function of cortisol concentration ranging from 1 fg to 1 µg in three electrode system. The magnitude of the electrochemical current response decreased while increasing the concentration of cortisol.

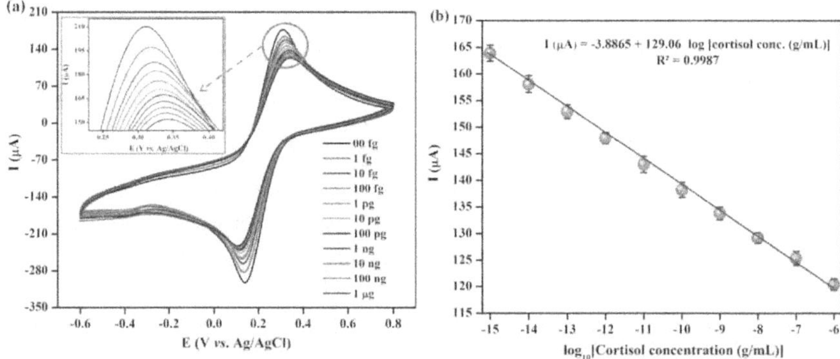

Fig. 4.14 (a) Electrochemical studies of BSA/Anti-C$_{mab}$/Fe$_2$O$_3$/CCY immunoelectrode as a function of cortisol concentration varied from 1 fg to 1 µg in PBS (10 mM, pH 7.0) and (b) Linear plot between electrochemical peak current response and logarithm of cortisol concentration

The formation of insulating immune complex between Anti-C_{mab} and cortisol was hindered electron transport which resulted in decreased current response which is shown in Fig. 4.14a. The calibration curve between the current response and logarithm of cortisol concentration has been plotted (Fig. 4.14b) in the range of 1 fg to 1 µg under optimized parameters. The linear regression equation (Eq. 4.3) was obtained as,

$$\Delta I \ (\mu A) = -3.886x + 129.06 \ [Cortisol \ conc. \ (g/mL); \ R^2 = 0.9987 \quad - - - (Eq. 4.3)$$

The detection limit of the fabricated BSA/Anti-C_{mab}/Fe$_2$O$_3$/CCY immunosensor was estimated as 0.005 fg using the standard equation (*Eq. 2.7*). The results were validated from three successive experiments (n=3) which indicated by the error bars (Fig. 4.14b).

4.4.5 Cortisol response studies of BSA/Anti-C$_{mab}$/Fe$_2$O$_3$/CCY immunoelectrode by DPV

Also, the electrochemical response of BSA/Anti-C_{mab}/Fe$_2$O$_3$/CCY immunoelectrode has been studied by DPV under similar condition used for CV. The DPV is sensitive analytical technique to study the electrochemical changes during biological reaction on the surface when the analyte concentration is very low [46]. Fig. 4.15a reveals the peak current of the BSA/Anti-C_{mab}/Fe$_2$O$_3$/CCY immunoelectrode decreased while increasing the cortisol concentration.

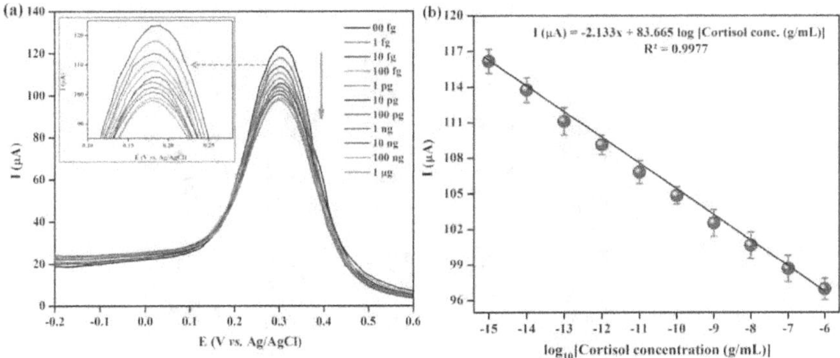

Fig. 4.15 (a) DPV analysis of the BSA/Anti-C_{mab}/Fe$_2$O$_3$/CCY immunoelectrode as a function of cortisol concentration varied from 1 fg to 1 µg in PBS (10 mM, pH 7.0) and (b) Linear plot between electrochemical peak current response and logarithm of cortisol concentration

This confirmed the effective formation of an immune-complex between antigen and antibody and the hindrance in electron transfer to the electrode due to the insulating behavior of cortisol. It is clear from Fig. 4.15b that linear curve attained between the logarithmic concentration of cortisol and peak current response revealed good linear range from 1 fg – 1 μg. The corresponding linear regression equation was obtained as (Eq. 4.4)

$$\Delta I\ (\mu A) = -2.133x + 83.66\ [Cortisol\ conc.\ (g/mL);\ R^2 = 0.9977 - - - (Eq.4.4)$$

As the DPV method is highly sensitive compared to CV in trace level analyte detection, the lower detection of limit was calculated from DPV outcomes as 0.003 fg/mL.

4.4.6 Interference studies

It is also important to evaluate how selectively and precisely the proposed sensing platform can detect cortisol in the presence of various interfering samples. The selectivity of the BSA/Anti-C_{mab}/Fe$_2$O$_3$/CCY immunoelectrode towards cortisol (100 ng/mL) have been tested with interference compounds especially cortisol analogous (100 ng/mL) such as progesterone, cortisone, BSA and cholesterol using CV technique in PBS (10 mM, pH 7.0).

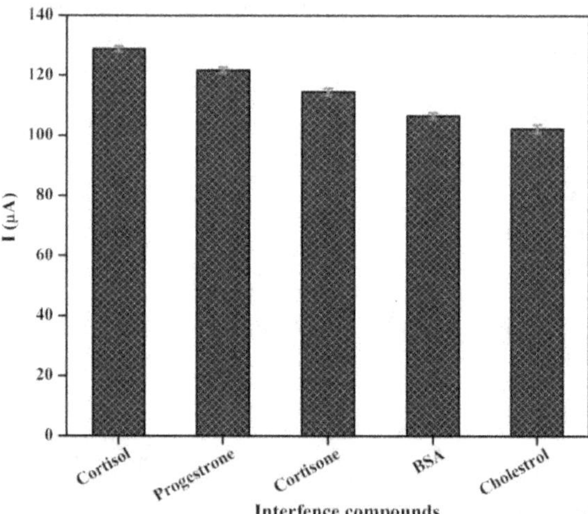

Fig. 4.16 Interference studies of BSA/Anti-C_{mab}/Fe$_2$O$_3$/CCY immunoelectrode towards Progesterone, Cortisone, Cholesterol and BSA with respect to cortisol (100 ng/mL) in PBS (10 mM, pH 7.0)

As shown in Fig. 4.16, the results exhibited a clear distinction of cortisol over competing species and decrement of electrochemical current response upto 5% to cortisol analogous. Although slight decrement in current response (<5%) was observed, no changes in the peak potentials of the immunosensor was observed when the interferents introduced into the cortisol solution. This confirmed that the sensing electrode material do not interact with the interferents. The high selectivity of the present sensor system was due to the use of monoclonal antibodies which forms specific immunocomplex binding sites with the target molecules. It can be concluded that the flexible and mediator free immunosensor electrode was highly selective towards cortisol estimation.

4.4.7 Stability, repeatability and reproducibility studies

To examine the repeatability of the BSA/Anti-C$_{mab}$/Fe$_2$O$_3$/CCY immunoelectrode, five separate electrodes were prepared and analyzed by CV technique. The average RSD of immunosensor was found to be 3.48 % from five measurements in presence of 100 ng/mL of cortisol. Additionally, the immunosensor was stored at 4 °C for 30 days and it was used to detect cortisol samples. The BSA/Anti-C$_{mab}$/Fe$_2$O$_3$/CCY immunosensor still retained 95.28 % of its response. The excellent stability of the immunosensor attributed to the strong interaction to the cortisol. The slight decrement in response might be due to the long-term deactivation of the immobilized biomolecules.

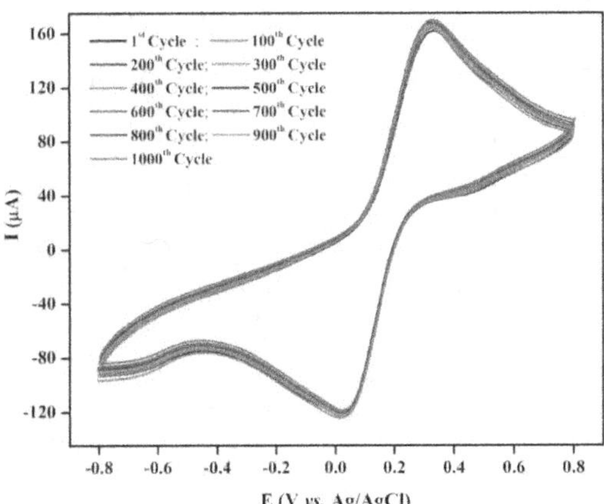

Fig. 4 17 The stability analysis of Fe$_2$O$_3$/CCY immunoelectrode for 1000 cycles in 10 mM PBS

Also, the stability of Fe$_2$O$_3$/CCY immunoelectrode was investigated by measuring the current response using CV for 1000 cycles in 10 mM PBS and the results are shown in Fig. 4.17 which assured the prepared immunosensor have agreeable reproducibility and stability.

4.4.8 Real sample analysis

We further examined the practicability of prepared immunosensor through analyzing real sweat samples analysis. Herein, CV method was used to detect the cortisol level in sweat. The RSD values of the proposed immunosensor corresponding to different sweat samples were ranging from 3.403 to 4.064 % and the recovery rates of the samples resulted between 98.67 % and 104.21%. The outcome values were validated using commercially available CLIA sensing method are shown in Fig. 4.18. A good correlation between the electrochemical measurements and CLIA results was observed. The results of both techniques are summarized in Table 4.1.

Table 4.1 Comparison of sweat cortisol estimated using chemiluminescence immunoassay and Fe$_2$O$_3$/CCY based electrochemical immunosensor

Samples	CLIA method (ng/mL)	Fe$_2$O$_3$/CCY immunosensor				
		Measured (ng/mL)*	Added (ng/mL)	Found (ng/mL)*	RSD (%)	Recovery (%)
1.	23	23.71	50	75.24	3.403	102.07
2.	24	27.81	50	77.51	3.874	99.62
3.	28	41.62	50	95.48	4.064	104.21
4.	46	44.20	50	96.43	3.548	102.36
5.	32	33.76	50	82.65	3.874	98.67

* The average value of three successive experiments

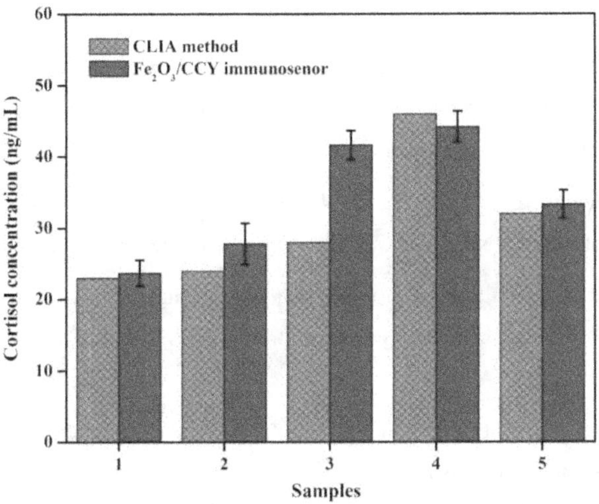

Fig. 4.18 Comparison graph of sweat cortisol estimated using chemiluminescence immunoassay and Fe₂O₃/CCY based electrochemical immunosensor

4.5 Conclusions

A highly sensitive and selective Fe₂O₃/CCY based flexible electrochemical sensor has been developed for the cortisol detection in sweat. The prepared immunosensor showed improved surface wettability, electrical conductivity and higher surface area which endorsed the improved sensing properties compared to previously reported SnO_2 and TiO_2 based immunosensors. The beneficial properties have resulted with higher detection range of 1 fg – 1 μg and detection limit of 0.005 fg/mL with the regression coefficient of 0.9987. The immunoelectrode identified with excellent selectivity to cortisol when compared to other cortisol analogous. Cortisol detection recovery was found in the range of 98.67 to 104.21% in human sweat samples. Response time of the immunosensor was 120 sec, and the sensing results were correlated well with chemiluminescence immunoassay and the negative cytotoxicity results also proved the applicability of the immunoelectrode. The proposed conductive yarn based system has great potential for commercialization as this platform could be readily integrated with fabrics and garments. With these results, further we have attempt to analyze the cortisol sensing ability of ZnO based immunosensor to obtain a standstill better performance and the results are discussed in next chapter.

References

1. L. Wang, X. Lu, C. Han, R. Lu, S. Yang, X. Song, Electrospun hollow cage-like α-Fe$_2$O$_3$ microspheres: synthesis, formation mechanism, and morphology-preserved conversion to Fe nanostructures, *CrystEngComm.*, **16** (2014) 10618–10623.

2. T. P. Almeida, M. Fay, Y. Zhu, P. D. Brown, Process map for the hydrothermal synthesis of α-Fe$_2$O$_3$ Nanorods, *J. Phys. Chem. C*, **113** (2009) 18689–18698.

3. D. Du and M. Cao, Ligand-assisted hydrothermal synthesis of hollow Fe$_2$O$_3$ urchin-like microstructures and their magnetic properties, *J. Phys. Chem. C*, **112** (2008) 10754-10758.

4. Z. H. Yang, Z. W. Li, J. Zhao, Y. H. Yang, Synthesis and enhanced microwave properties of uniform hollow Fe nanospheres and their core–shell silica nanocomposites, *RSC Adv.*, **4** (2014) 9457-9462.

5. C. Pulgarin and J. Kiwi, Iron oxide-mediated degradation, photodegradation, and biodegradation of aminophenols, *Langmuir*, **11** (1995) 519-526.

6. C. Wu, P.Yin, X. Zhu, C. O. Yang, Y. Xie, Synthesis of Hematite (α-Fe$_2$O$_3$) nanorods: Diameter-size and shape effects on their applications in magnetism, lithium ion battery and gas sensors, *J. Phys. Chem. B*, **110** (2006) 17806-17812.

7. V. Polshettiwar, R. Luque, A. Fihri, H. B. Zhu, M. Bouhrara, J. M. Basset, Magnetically recoverable nanocatalysts. *Chem. Rev.*, **111** (2011) 3036–3075.

8. H. O. Finklea, Semiconductor electrodes, Publisher: Elsevier (1988) *ISBN 0-444-42926-3.*

9. A. Qurashi, Z. H. Zhong, M. W. Alam, Synthesis and photocatalytic properties of α-Fe$_2$O$_3$ nanoellipsoids, *Solid State Sci.*, **12** (2010) 1516–1519.

10. S. W. Cao, Y. J. Zhu, G. F. Cheng, Y. H. Huang, Preparation and photocatalytic property of α-Fe$_2$O$_3$ hollow core shell hierarchical nanostructures, *J. Phys. Chem. Sol.*, **71** (2010) 1680–1683.

11. W. Wang, J. Y. Howe, B. Gu, Structure and morphology evolution of Hematite (α-Fe$_2$O$_3$) nanoparticles in forced hydrolysis of ferric chloride, *J. Phys. Chem. C,* **112** (2008) 9203-9208.

12. X. Yang and L. Li, Controlled synthesis of single-crystalline α-Fe$_2$O$_3$ micro/ nanoparticles from the complex precursor of FeCl$_3$ and methyl orange, *Nanotechnology,* **21** (2010) 355602.

13. B. Jia and L. Gao, Growth of Well-defined cubic hematite single crystals: oriented aggregation and ostwald ripening, *Cryst. Growth Des.,* **8** (2008) 1372-1376.

14. J. Lu, D. Chen, X. Jiao, Fabrication, characterization, and formation mechanism of hollow spindle-like hematite via a solvothermal process, *J. Colloid Interface Sci.,* **303** (2006) 437-443.

15. Y. Fu, J. Chen, H. Zhang, Synthesis of Fe$_2$O$_3$ nanowires by oxidation of iron, *Chem. Phys Lett.,* **350** (2001) 491-494.

16. D. L. Huber, Synthesis, properties and applications of iron nanoparticles, *Small,* **5** (2005) 482-501

17. D. V. Talapin, J. S. Lee, M. V. Kovalenko, E. V. Shevchenko, Prospects of colloidal nanocrystals for electronic and optoelectronic applications, *Chem. Rev.,* **110** (2009) 389-458.

18. N. Pailhe, J. Majimel, S. Pechev, P. Gravereau, M. Gaudon, A. Demourgues, Investigation of nanocrystallized α-Fe$_2$O$_3$ prepared by a precipitation process, *J. Phys. Chem. C,* **112** (2008) 19217−19223.

19. X. D. Xu, R. G. Cao, S. Jeong, J. Cho, Spindle-like mesoporous α-Fe$_2$O$_3$ anode material prepared from MOF template for high-rate lithium batteries. *Nano Lett.,* **12** (2012) 4988−4991.

20. W. Hamd, S. Cobo, J. Fize, G. Baldinozzi, W. Schwartz, M. Reymermier, A. Pereira, M. Fontecave, V. Artero, C. Laberty-Robert C. Sanchez, Mesoporous α-Fe$_2$O$_3$ thin films synthesized via the sol-gel process for light-driven water oxidation. *Phys. Chem. Chem. Phys.,* **14** (2012) 13224−13232.

21. M. Saleem, M. F. Al-Kuhaili, S. M. A. Durrani, I. A. Bakhtiari, Characterization of nanocrystalline α-Fe$_2$O$_3$ thin films grown by reactive evaporation and oxidation of iron. *Phys. Scr.*, **85** (2012) 055802−055802.

22. P. S. Shinde, G. H. Go, W. J. Lee, Facile growth of Hierarchical hematite (α-Fe$_2$O$_3$) nanopetals on FTO by pulse reverse electrodeposition for photoelectrochemical Water Splitting, *J. Mater. Chem*, **22** (2012) 10469−10471.

23. H. G. Cha, C. W. Kim, Y. H. Kim, M. H. Jung, E. S. Ji, B. K. Das, J. C. Kim, Y. S. Kang, Preparation and characterization of α-Fe$_2$O$_3$ nanorod-thin film by metal-organic chemical vapor deposition, *Thin solid films*, **517** (2009) 1853−1856.

24. D. N. Lei, M. Zhang, B. H. Qu, L. B. Chen, Y. G. Wang, E. D. Zhang, Z. Xu, Q. H. Li, T. H. Wang, α-Fe$_2$O$_3$ Nanowall Arrays: hydrothermal preparation, growth mechanism and excellent rate performances for lithium ion batteries, *Nanoscale*, **4** (2012) 3422− 3426.

25. J. Ma, J. Lian, X. Duan, X. Liu, W. Zheng, α-Fe$_2$O$_3$: Hydrothermal synthesis, magnetic and electrochemical properties, *J. Phys. Chem. C*, **114** (2010) 10671−10676.

26. X. Wang, M. Zhang, E. Liua, F. He, C. Shi, C. He, J. Li, N. Zhao, Three-dimensional core-shell Fe$_2$O$_3$@carbon/carbon cloth as binder-free anode for the high-performance lithium-ion batteries, *Appl. Surf. Sci.*, **390** (2016) 350–356.

27. L. Ji, O. Toprakci, M. Alcoutlabi, Y. Yao, Y. Li, S. Zhang, B. Guo, Z. Lin, X. Zhang, α-Fe$_2$O$_3$ Nanoparticle-loaded carbon nanofibers as stable and high-capacity anodes for rechargeable lithium-ion batteries, *ACS Appl. Mater. Interfaces*, **4** (2012) 2672−2679.

28. K. P. O. Mahesh, I. Shown, L. C. Chen, K. H. Chen, Y. Tai, Flexible sensor for dopamine detection fabricated by the direct growth of α-Fe$_2$O$_3$ nanoparticles on carbon cloth, *Appl. Surf. Sci.*, **427** (2018) 387–395.

29. S. K. Arya, A. Dey, S. Bhansali, Polyaniline protected gold nanoparticles based mediator free electrochemical cortisol biosensor and label free electrochemical cortisol biosensor, *Biosens. Bioelectron.*, **28** (2011) 166 − 173.

30. X. F. Qu, Q. Z. Yao, G. T. Zhou, S. Q. Fu, J. L. Huang, Formation of hollow magnetite microspheres and their evolution into durian-like architectures, *J. Phys. Chem. C*, **114** (2010) 8734–8740.

31. C. Sun, S. Chen, Z. Li, Controllable synthesis of Fe_2O_3-carbon fiber composites via a facile sol-gel route as anode materials for lithium ion batteries, *Appl. Surf. Sci.,* **427** (2018) 476–484.

32. X. Wang, M. Zhang, E. Liu, F. He, C. Shi, C. He, J. Li, N. Zhao, Three-dimensional core-shell Fe_2O_3@carbon/carbon cloth as binder-free anode for the high-performance lithium-ion batteries, *Appl. Surf. Sci.,* **390** (2016) 350–356.

33. J. Song, Q. Yuan, X. Liu, D. Wang, F. Fu, W. Yang, Combination of nitrogen plasma modification and waterborne polyurethane treatment of carbon fiber paper used for electric heating of wood floors, *Bioresources,* **10** (2015) 5820-5829.

34. Y. Zou, J. Kan, Y. Wang, Fe_2O_3-graphene rice-on-sheet nanocomposite for high and fast lithium ion storage, *J. Phys. Chem. C,* **115** (2011) 20747–20753.

35. Q. Qiu, H. Huang, H. Genuino, N. Opembe, L. Stafford, S. Dharmarathna, S. L. Suib, Microwave-assisted hydrothermal synthesis of nanosized α-Fe_2O_3 for catalysts and adsorbents, *J. Phys. Chem. C,* **115** (2011) 19626–19631.

36. H. F. Ma, T. T. Chen, Y. Luo, F. Y. Kong, D. H. Fan, H. L. Fang, W. Wang, Electrochemical determination of dopamine using octahedral SnO_2 nanocrystals bound to reduced graphene oxide nanosheets, *Microchim. Acta,* **182** (2015) 2001–2007.

37. S. Madhu, P. Manickam, M. Pierre, S. Bhansali, P. Nagamony, V. Chinnuswamy, Nanostructured SnO_2 integrated conductive fabrics as binder-free electrode for neurotransmitter detection, *Sens. Actuators A Phys,* **269** (2018) 401–411.

38. P. Manivel, D. Mangalaraj, M. Dhakshnamoorthy, A. Balamurugan, N. Ponpandian, C. Viswanathan, Conducting polyaniline-graphene oxide fibrous nanocomposites: preparation, characterization and simultaneous electrochemical detection of ascorbic acid, dopamine and uric acid, *RSC Adv.,* **3** (2013) 14428-14437.

39. Z. Jian, B. Zhao, P. Liu, F. Li, M. Zheng, M. Chen, Y. Shi, H. Zhou, Fe_2O_3 nanocrystals anchored onto graphene nanosheets as the anode material for low-cost sodium-ion batteries, *Chem. Commun.,* **50** (2014) 1215 - 1217.

40. L. F. Chen, Z. Y. Yu, X. Ma, Z. Y. Li, S. H. Yu, In situ hydrothermal growth of ferric oxides on carbon cloth for low-cost and scalable high-energy-density supercapacitors, *Nano Energy,* **9** (2014) 345–354.

41. G. Zhou, D. W. Wang, L. C. Yin, N. Li, F. Li, H. M. Cheng, Oxygen bridges between NiO nanosheets and graphene for improvement of lithium storage, *ACS Nano,* **6** (2012) 3214-3223.

42. T. Li, H. Yu, L. Zhi, W. Zhang, L. Dang, Z. H. Liu, Z. Lei, Facile electrochemical fabrication of porous Fe_2O_3 nanosheets for flexible asymmetric supercapacitor, *J. Phys. Chem. C,* **121**, (2017) 18982-18991

43. M. Reyssat, J. M. Yeomans, D. Quére, Impalement of fakir drops, *Europhys Lett.,* **81** (2008) 26006 (1-5).

44. H. S. Ahn, H. Kim, J. M. Kim, S. C. Park, J. M. Kim, J. Kim, M. H. Kim, Controllable pore size of three dimensional self-assembled foam-like graphene and its wettability, *Carbon,* **64** (2013) 27-34.

45. A. Kaushik, A. Vasudev, S. K. Arya, S. Bhansali, Mediator and label free estimation of stress biomarker using electrophoretically deposited Ag at AgO-polyaniline hybrid nanocomposite, *Biosens. Bioelectron.,* **50** (2013) 35–41.

46. R. Sriramprabha, M. Divagar, D. Mangalaraj, N. Ponpandian, C. Viswanathan, Formulation of SnO_2/graphene nanocomposite modified electrode for synergetic electrochemical detection of dopamine, *Adv. Mater. Lett.,* **6** (2015) 973-977.

Chapter V

Vertically Aligned ZnO Nanorods Integrated Carbon Fibers Functionalized with Antibodies for Highly Sensitive Cortisol Detection

Highlights

> 1D ZnO nanorods (ZnO NRs) were uniformly deposited onto CCY surface by hydrothermal method at controlled conditions.

> Integration of ZnO NRs onto the CCY were characterized using XRD, FE-SEM, HR-TEM and EDS mapping analysis.

> EDC/NHS chemistry was used to immobilize anti-cortisol antibodies onto the ZnO-NRs/CCY electrodes.

> The detection limit of the immunosensor was found to be 0.45 fg, well below the physiological concentrations of cortisol.

> Sweat cortisol levels measured using immunosensors are correlated well with commercial CILA method.

Graphical illustration of immobilization and electrochemical immunosensing of cortisol on hydrothermally derived ZnO NRs/CCY with possible redox mechanism

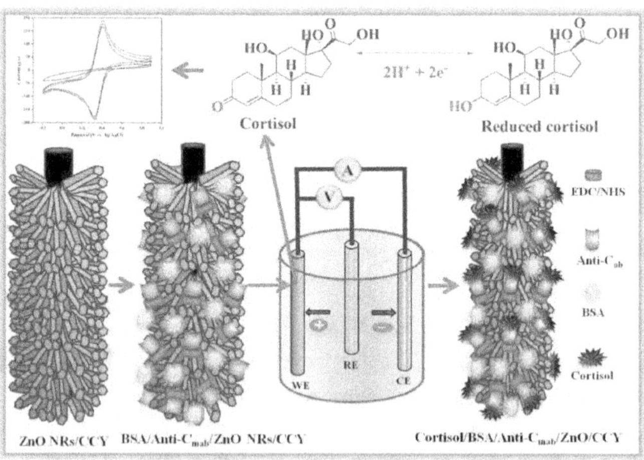

5.1 Introduction

Integration of the conductive inorganic nanostructures onto flexible materials such as paper, fabrics and plastics will empower strategy of novel functional materials such as smart clothing with sensing and wearable electronics, renewable energy systems protection capabilities and portable and flexible photovoltaic devices [1-4]. Among the semiconducting metal oxides, nanostructured zinc oxide (ZnO) is an exceptionally important material to study, due to its attractive physical properties such as wide band gap (3.37 eV) and large exaction binding energy (60 meV) at room temperature [5, 6]. ZnO nanostructures are proved to be biocompatible and low-toxic have high catalytic efficiency and chemical stability in physiological environments [7, 8]. Because of this unique optical and electrical properties, ZnO has potential applications in solar cells, UV lasers, light-emitting diodes (LED)], field-effect transistors and electrochemical sensors [9-14].

The tremendous interest in ZnO is due to its unique ability of possessing structure dependent properties. Therefore, the design and synthesis of ZnO nanomaterials with different structures are got specific attention. ZnO nanostructures with preferred morphologies such as nanorods (NRs), nanoflakes (NFs), nanowalls, nanobelts and quantum dots have been synthesized and used as immobilizing matrix in the preparation of biosensors for the detection of physiologically relevant biomarkers such as cholesterol, galactose, glucose [15-20]. These nanostructures have inimitable advantages which make ZnO has one of the most promising materials for biosensor applications [21].

ZnO NRs, among the one-dimensional (1D) nanostructures, boast high surface-to-volume ratio and high electron mobility [22] provides a direct, stable pathway for rapid electron transport and they have emerged as a very promising material for immobilization of biomolecules without the aid of electron mediators used in immunosensors [23-26]. These sensors have demonstrated high stability, better sensitivity, fast response time and excellent selectivity. Specifically, metal-oxide nanorods could play a vital role in the development of these functional materials due to their ease of synthesis, morphology, crystallinity, quantum confinement effects and directional mobility of charge carriers [27]. The hexagonal wurtzite crystal structure of ZnO is shown in Fig. 5.1.

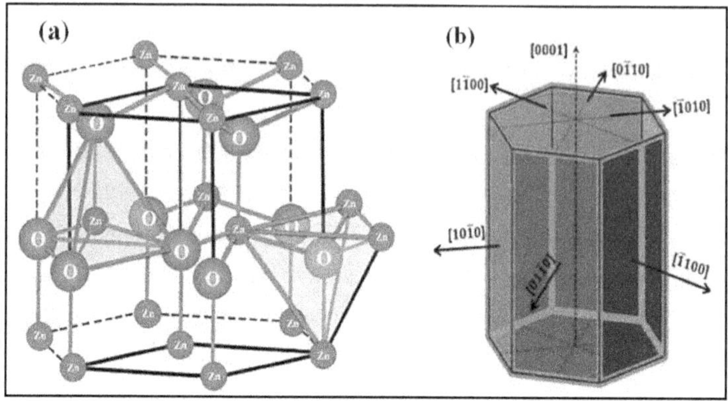

Fig. 5.1 (a) Hexagonal wurtzite crystal structure of ZnO and (b) Hexagonal prism of ZnO crystal showing different crystallographic faces

Z. Zhao *et al.*, effectively used the ZnO nanostructure as binder free electrode material for the enzyme immobilization for the sensitive detection of glucose using primarily amperometric based sensing techniques [28]. Wang *et al.*, used ZnO nanocombs on gold electrodes functionalized with Nafion for glucose detection. The sensor demonstrated with detection limit of 3.6 mg/mL glucose in PBS [29]. Kong *et al.*, described the amperometric enzymatic detection of glucose with the detection limit of 0.02 mg/dL in PBS using ZnO nanotubes immobilized with glucose oxidase [30]. Pradhan *et al.*, demonstrated the growth of ZnO nanowires on gold plated polyester flexible substrate and enzymatic glucose detection with a detection limit of 9 mg/mL [31].

Vabbina *et al.*, (2015) have synthesized 1D ZnO NRs and two-dimensional (2D) ZnO nanoflakes (ZnO-NF) Au substrates using sonochemical method and used as immobilization matrix for fabricating cortisol sensors. Anti-cortisol antibodies were immobilized onto the ZnO nanostructures for detection of cortisol using electrochemical technique. The ZnO NRs showed a sensitivity of 11.86 mA/M while the ZnO-NFs showed the sensitivity of 7.74 mA/M for cortisol detection. Both the platform exhibited the lowest detection limit of 1 pM which is 100 times better than the conventional ELISA method [7]. Munje *et al.*, (2017) demonstrated a flexible and wearable electrochemical biosensor for the combinatorial label-free detection of glucose and cortisol in human sweat. The novel device comprises of stacked metal/metal-oxide (Au/ZnO) thin films within porous polyamide substrates for low-volume ultrasensitive impedance-based electrochemical detection of glucose and cortisol. The reliable LOD of 0.1 mg/dL in human sweat was achieved [32]. Usha *et al.,* (2016) developed a fiber optic salivary cortisol sensor using a contemporary method of lossy mode resonance and molecular imprinting of nanocomposites of ZnO and polypyrrole. The sensor response was linear up to the concentration range 10^{-6} g/mL of cortisol prepared using artificial saliva. The sensor also showed a lowest detection limit of 25.9 fg/mL [33].

Carbon cloth, is a carbonous materials, has good conductivity, excellent flexibility, unique mechanical strength, which is widely applied in electrochemical fields compared to other carbon nanomaterials such as graphene, activated carbon, and porous carbon, etc. In recent years, plenty of transition metal oxide/hydroxide with carbon cloth has been used to improve the sensing performance in electrochemical sensors and energy storage [34, 35]. The preparation of ZnO NRs on CCY, carbon yarn covered with 3D vertical ZnO nanorods allows for considerably large contact area with the electrolyte and more surface active sites available for antigen-antibody interaction in the cortisol detection. There are no reports available on cortisol detection using the vertically aligned ZnO NRs on carbon yarn.

This *chapter V* discuss the preparation of vertically grown/alligned ZnO NRs on flexible CCY surface (designated as ZnO NRs/CCY) to prepare a binder free electrode by a facile and scalable hydrothermal method. For sensitive cortisol estimation, Anti-C$_{mab}$ was immobilized on ZnO NRs matrix via electrostatic interaction. The electron transfer properties of antibody functionalized ZnO NRs upon binding with various concentrations of cortisol were studied using electrochemical techniques. CV and DPV studies revealed that the sensor (Anti-C$_{mab}$ /ZnO/NRs/CCY) showed high sensitivity and lowest detection for cortisol. For real sample analysis, the developed immunosensors were tested with human sweat cortisol and the results were validated using commercial CILA method.

5.2 Materials and methods

5.2.1 Chemicals and reagents

All chemicals were of analytical grade and were used without further purification. Zinc nitrate hexahydrate [$Zn(NO_3)_2.6H_2O$], hexamethylenetetramine (HMTA) ($C_6H_{12}N_4$)

were obtained from Sigma Aldrich, India. Carbon cloth was purchased from Vinpro tech, Hyderabad. All other chemical like cortisol and its analogous used for electrochemical sensing given in chapter II.). All aqueous solutions were prepared with DD water.

5.2.2 Preparation of ZnO seed layer on CCY substrate

The ZnO hydrothermal synthesis technique requires a pre-deposited ZnO seed layer on top of the fibers; providing initiation seeds for growing the uniform ZnO nanorods [36]. The dimensions and morphology of the grown ZnO nanorods can be tuned by employing different concentrations of chemicals inside the solution, time of the growth, solution temperature by which the initiation seeds were pre-deposited [37, 38]. The carbon yarn substrate was ultrasonically washed with acetone, water and ethanol for 30 min individually finally treated under 90 °C for 12 hrs prior to use.

The seeding process was performed by RF magnetron sputtering (Huttenger instrument) with Ar^+ as working gas and O_2 as reactive gas in 1:5 (sccm) ratios. The Zn metal used as target in the working pressure of 10^{-2} m.bar and RF power of 150 W for depositing a thin layer of ZnO as a seed layer on CCY for 30 min.

5.2.3 Growth of vertically aligned ZnO NRs array on CCY surface

ZnO was initially coated on bare CCY by sputtering process because of uniform growth followed by the hydrothermally grown ZnO NRs. The equimolar ratio of 5 mM HMTA and $Zn(NO_3)_2.6H_2O$ were dissolved in 80 mL of DD water. The resulting suspension was transferred into a Teflon-lined stainless-steel autoclave and the seed layers coated on multiple CCYs were hanged in the reaction solution. The hydrothermal treatments were carried out at 90 °C for 6 hrs. After that, the autoclave was allowed to cool down gradually to the room temperature. Finally, the ZnO NRs coated CCY removed from the growth solution and washed with DD water and ethanol for several times and dried in air at room temperature.

5.2.4 Immobilization of Anti-C_{mab} on ZnO NRs/CCY

For the preparation of ZnO NRs immunosensor, 80 µL of Anti-C_{mab} was covalently immobilized via electrostatic interaction of due to the difference in IEPs of ZnO (9.5) and Anti-C_{mab} (4.5) using EDC and NHS chemistry. The ZnO NRs/CCY electrodes were incubated with Anti-C$_{mab}$ for 120 mins followed by PBS (10 mM, pH 7.0) washing to remove any unbound molecules. The non-binding sites of Anti-C$_{mab}$/ZnO NRs/CCY immunoelectrode were blocked by immobilizing 50 µL of BSA for 30 mins. After washed by PBS the immunoelectrodes and dried at room temperature. The prepared BSA/Anti-C$_{mab}$/ZnO NRs/CCY immunoelectrodes were stored at 4 °C when not in use.

5.2.5 Possible growth mechanism of ZnO NRs on CCY

The aqueous solutions of Zn(NO$_3$)$_2$.6H$_2$O and HMTA can produce the following chemical reactions. The concentration of HMTA plays a vital role for the formation of ZnO NRs. Since (OH)$^-$ is strongly related to the reaction that produces nanostructures. Literatures reported that amine can be an effective surfactant; being a non-polar chelating agent, it covers the non-polar planes (100) and (110) of ZnO and consequently facilitates the growth of ZnO nanostructures along the [001] c-axis (anisotropic growth) [39, 40]. However, higher rate of Zn super saturation will offer the growth along multiple planes (isotropic growth). Rate of Zn supersaturation used to determine the morphology of the ZnO nanostructures as lower Zn supersaturation promotes 1D, anisotropic nanorods growth, and increase in Zn supersaturation favors for 3D, isotropic growth along multiple planes.

Initially, owing to decomposition of Zn(NO$_3$)$_2$.6H$_2$O and HMTA at an elevated temperature, OH was introduced in Zn^{2+} aqueous solution and their concentration increased and given in following equations (Eq. 5.1 to Eq. 5.7)

$$Zn(NO_3)_2 \rightarrow Zn^{2+} + 2NO_3^- \quad -------------(Eq.5.1)$$

$$(CH_2)_6N_4 + 6H_2O \rightarrow 6HCHO + 4NH_3 \quad --------(Eq.5.2)$$

$$NH_4OH \leftrightarrow NH_3 + H_2O \quad ----------------(Eq.5.3)$$

$$Zn^{2+} + 4NH_3 \leftrightarrow Zn[(NH_3)_4]^{2+} \quad -----------(Eq.5.4)$$

$$2H_2O \leftrightarrow H_3O + OH^- \quad ------------------(Eq.5.5)$$

$$Zn^{2+} + 2OH^- \leftrightarrow Zn(OH)_2 \quad --------------(Eq.5.6)$$

$$Zn(OH)_2 \rightarrow ZnO + H_2O \quad ---------------(Eq.5.7)$$

The separated colloidal $Zn(OH)_2$ clusters in solution will act partly as nuclei for the growth of ZnO nanorods. During the hydrothermal growth process, the $Zn(OH)_2$ dissolved completely by applied temperature. When the concentrations of Zn^{2+} and OH ions reached the critical value of supersaturation of the ZnO, the fine ZnO nuclei form spontaneously in the aqueous complex solution. When the solution was reached supersaturated state, the nucleation got initiated. Subsequently, the ZnO nanoparticles combine together to reduce the interfacial free energy. This was because the molecules at the surface would have been energetically less stable than the already well ordered and packed in the interior. Since the (001) face has higher symmetry than the other faces growing along the c-axis [(0001) direction], it is the typical growth plane on the surface of the CCY. The nucleation determines the surface-to-volume ratio of the ZnO nanorods. Then incorporation of growth units into crystal lattice of the nanorods formed by the dehydration of $Zn(OH)_2$ to yield ZnO reaction [41, 42].

5.3 Results and Discussion

5.3.1 XRD analysis of CCY and ZnO NRs/CCY

The direct growth of ZnO NRs on the CCY was successfully carried out using the simple hydrothermal method. The crystal structure of CCY and ZnO NRs/CCY is confirmed by the XRD results which are shown in Fig. 5.2. The XRD profile of the CCY shows two broad shoulder peaks at 26.0° and 43.6°, which correspond to the (002) and (100) planes of hexagonal graphitic carbon. The ZnO NRs/CCY showed major sharp peaks around 31.79°, 34.42°, 36.25°, 47.54°, 56.60°, 63.86°, 66.37°, 68.2°, 69.2°, 72.2° and 77.2°, which attributed from the diffraction planes (110), (002), (101), (102), (110), (002), (200), (112), (201) and (104) of ZnO NRs along with carbon peaks. All of these diffraction peaks are closely matched the hexagonal wurtzite phase of the reference profile of JCPDS No.: 36-1451. The ZnO crystal in hexagonal wurtzite-type structure, which is thermodynamically stable at ambient conditions, may be composed of alternating planes composed of four-fold coordinated O^{2-} and Zn^{2+} ions stacked alternately along the c-axis. There are no other characteristic peaks revealing the existence of crystalline phases, thus confirming the formation of pure ZnO NRs on CCY [43, 44].

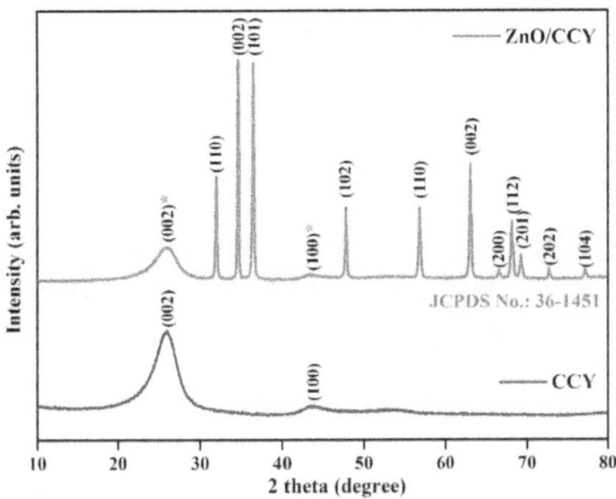

Fig. 5.2 X-ray diffraction patterns of CCY and ZnO NRs/CCY

Crystallite size of ZnO was obtained by Scherrer's formula. β selected diffraction peak corresponding to plane (101) and θ is the Bragg angle obtained from 2θ value corresponding to maximum intensity peak in XRD pattern (Fig. 5.2). The crystallite size obtained was ~ 12 nm.

5.3.2 FI-IR spectra of CCY and ZnO NRs/CCY

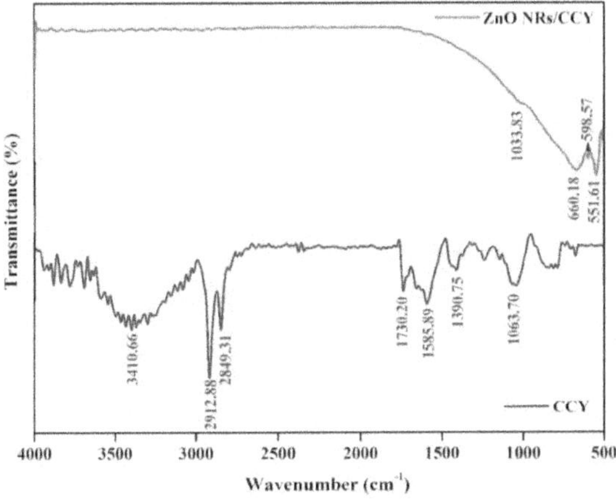

Fig. 5.3 FTIR spectra of CCY and ZnO NRs/CCY

FTIR spectra (Fig. 5.3) were attained to explore the condition of functional groups upon samples of CCY and ZnO NRs/CCY. The peaks at 2912 and 2849 cm^{-1} of sample CCY indicate CH$_2$ asymmetric stretching and -CH$_2$ symmetric stretching vibrations, respectively. A strong peak at 1390 cm^{-1} corresponded to the C-C bond stretching. A characteristic peak at 1585 cm^{-1} corresponds to C=C bond. The stretching vibration peak at 1063 and 1033 cm^{-1} were assigned to C-O bond and the peak at 1730 cm^{-1} corresponds to C=O group of carbon in the CCY and ZnO NRs/CCY. The broad peak at 3410 cm^{-1} for CCY was -OH stretching vibration might due to small amounts of absorbed water [45].

A strong peak arouses at 551, 598 and 660 cm^{-1} is the characteristic of stretching vibration in ZnO in ZnO NRs/CCY. In the FT-IR spectrum of the ZnO NRs/CCY showed all of peaks appeared at the spectra of ZnO and CCY just the intensity of peaks was comparatively low. This may be due to the dense and uniform coating of ZnO nanorods on carbon yarn surface [46, 47].

5.3.3 RAMAN spectra of CCY and ZnO NRs/CCY

The microstructure of CCY and the ZnO NRs / CCY were evaluated using Raman spectroscopy. The Fig. 5.4 shows a representative Raman spectrum of CCY and it has two peaks at 1355 and 1592 cm^{-1}, which correspond to the defected sp^2 carbon "D-band" (A$_{1g}$) and the in-plane vibrations of the graphite "G-band" (E$_{2g}$) respectively.

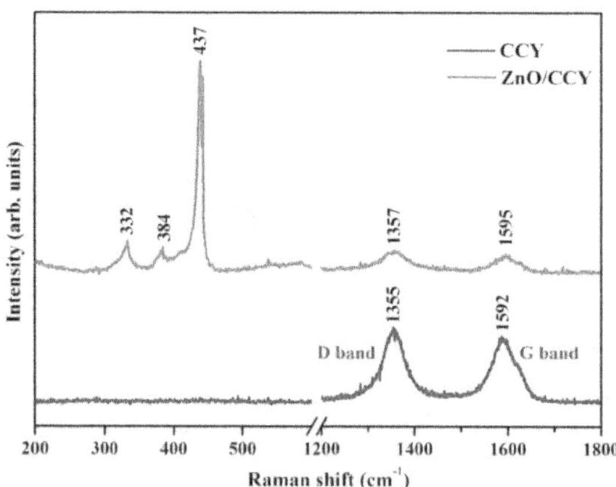

Fig. 5.4 Raman spectra of CCY and ZnO NRs/CCY

Furthermore, the Raman spectrum of ZnO NRs/CCY showed the characteristic peaks located at 332, 384, 437, 1357 and 1595 cm^{-1}. The peak at 437 cm^{-1} was corresponding to the E_2 mode of ZnO NRs which attributed from the hexagonal wurtzite phase. Another peak at 332 cm^{-1} could be attributed to the second-order Raman spectrum arising from zone-boundary phonons of ZnO. The D and G bands in ZnO NRs/CCY might merged with the ZnO peaks because their resultant intensity was very small in comparison to the ZnO peaks. The Raman spectra results further confirmed that the prepared ZnO did not possess any other impurity phases and the interfacial bonding of the composite. The results were also in good agreement with the XRD results, confirmed the formation of the hexagonal phase of ZnO [47-49].

5.3.4 Morphological and compositional analysis of CCY and ZnO NRs/CCY

The surface morphology and compositions of CCY and ZnO NRs/CCY were characterized by FE-SEM equipped with EDS and the results were shown in Fig. 5.5 (a-f). The FE-SEM image (Fig. 5.5 a&b) of CCY showed a smooth and uniform surface of the yarn along the complete length. Fig. 5.5 (c-f) shows the magnified FE-SEM image ZnO NRs coated CCY obtained after undergoing a typical sputtering process. The grown ZnO NRs are pointing outwards from the fiber surface and forming in well arrayed pattern. The estimated maximum length and diameter of the ZnO NRs is 800-900 nm and 100 nm respectively. It revealed that the CCY is fully coated by uniform and dense ZnO nanorods. Also, Fig. 5.5f shows that each nanorod exhibited a hexagonal end surface.

Furthermore, the EDS spectrum of the ZnO NRs directly grown on CCY proved the presence of the Zn (73.27%) and O (17.88%) elements along with C (8.84%) in the sample, as shown in Fig. 5.6a. The EDS elemental mapping (Fig. 3.6b) analysis of ZnO NRs/CCY effectively proved the existence and uniform distribution of Zn, O and C in the ZnO NRs/CCY which indicates the high purity ZnO NRs grown on CCY.

Furthermore, investigation the structure of ZnO NRs, HR-TEM and associated electron diffraction are displayed in Fig. 5.7. The low-magnification TEM image of ZnO NRs is shown in Fig. 5.7a, which indicates the morphology of single nanorod and the result was in good accordance with the FE-SEM results. Fig. 5.7b exhibits the selected-area electron diffraction (SAED) pattern was indicating the high single-crystalline property of ZnO NRs and that could be indexed to the hexagonal ZnO phase which can be agreed with the XRD results in Fig. 5.2.

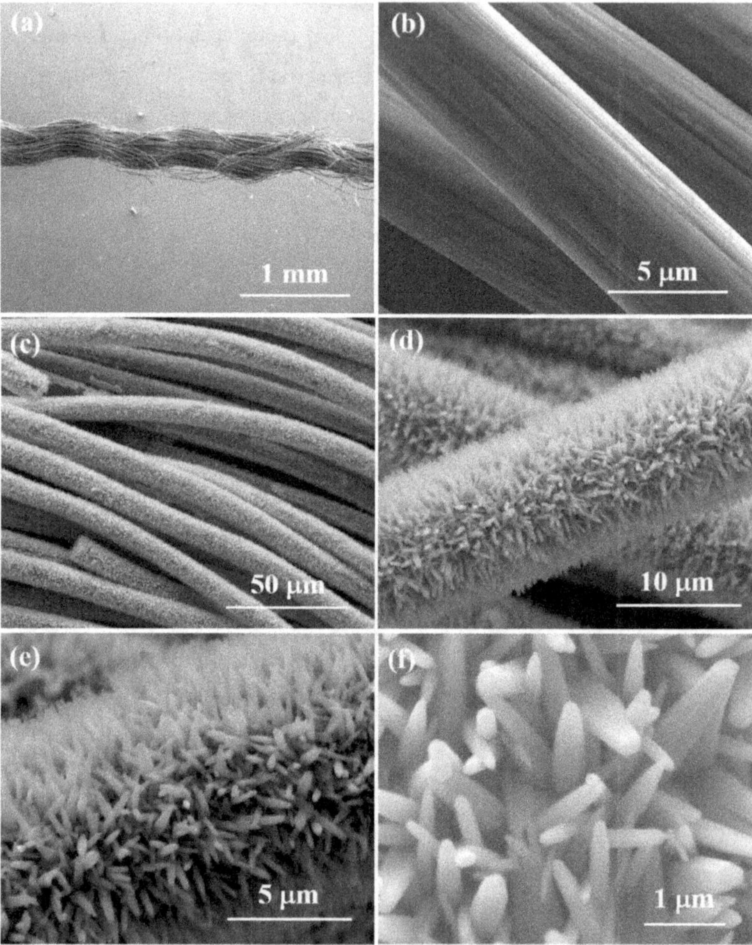

Fig. 5.5 FESEM images of (a & b) bare CCY and (c–f) ZnO NRs/CCY with different magnifications

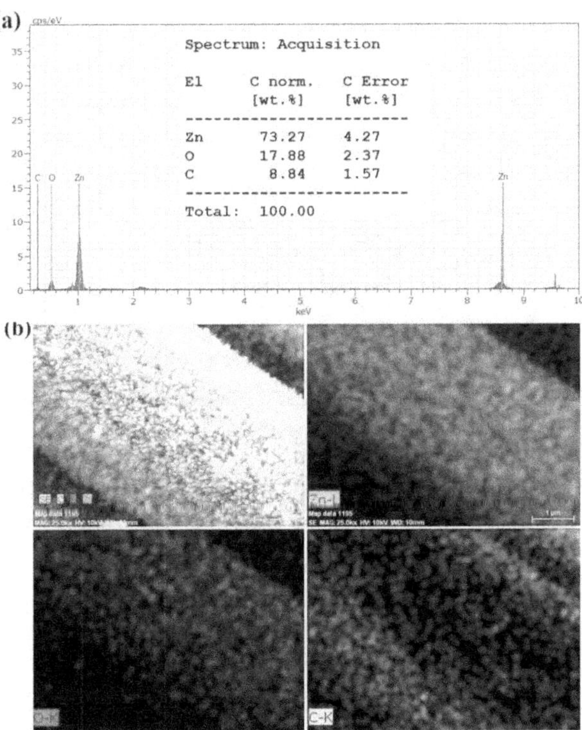

Fig. 5.6 (a) EDS spectra ZnO NRs /CCY and (B) corresponding FESEM image and EDS mapping of ZnO NRs /CCY

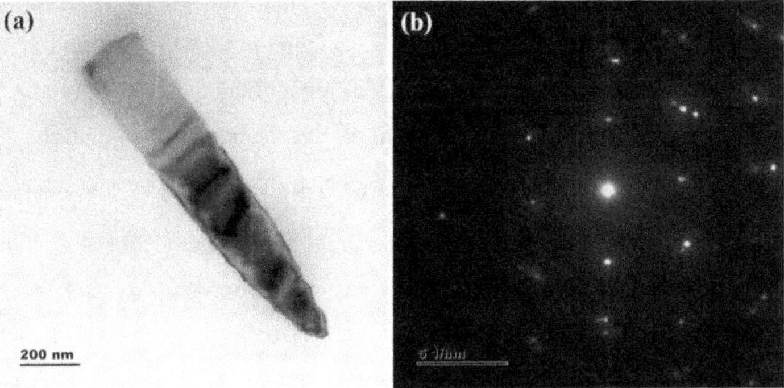

Fig. 5.7 (a) HRTEM image and (b) SAED pattern of ZnO NRs

5.3.5 Electrical and mechanical properties of CCY and ZnO NRs/CCY

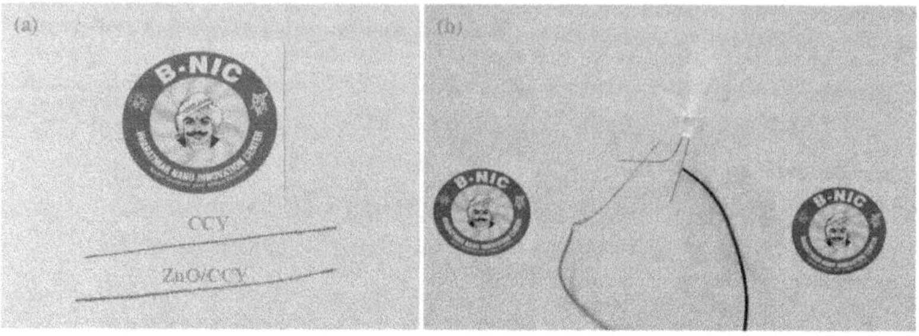

Fig. 5.8 Photographs of CCY-ZnO NRs/CCY; (a) Comparison of the pure CCY and ZnO NRs/CCY and (b) Demonstration of LED emission with the current passing through ZnO NRs coated CCY

In order to investigate the electrical properties, the electrical resistance of 5 cm long CCY and ZnO NRs anchored CCY were measured. The resistance of the ZnO NRs/CCY (54.3 ± 1.2 Ω) increased when compared to the bare CCY (36 ± 1 Ω). Also, the conductivity of ZnO NRs/CCY was demonstrated by powering an LED device connected to a battery as shown in Fig. 5.8. The amount of ZnO NRs deposited on the CCY (5 cm length) is around 1.5 mg.

The mechanical properties of CCY and ZnO NRs coated CCY were investigated tensile, elongation and elastic modulus tests. The ultimate strength measured for ZnO NRs was found to be 38.40 MPa. This value was higher than the bare CCY (20.10 MPa). These suggest the strength of the fiber was enhanced because of the ZnO NRs array was covered on the entire surface of CCY. Also, elongation and young's modulus of the ZnO NRs/CCY (6.82 % and 57.17 MPa) were improved after ZnO incorporation (7.53 % and 37.17 MPa). The mechanical strength of the ZnO NRs/CCY is higher than that of the pure CCY due to a densification, and stronger adhesion of the fibers to each other by the material.

5.3.6 Specific and assessable surface area of CCY and ZnO NRs/CCY electrode

The ZnO NRs/CCY sample has a larger specific surface area (138.116 m^2/g) compared to the uncoated CCY which was ascribed to its featured morphology and the improved vertically aligned ZnO NRs facilitated by the carbon surface. Visibly, it was clear that uniform coating of ZnO nanorods arrays on CCY possesses much higher specific surface area as compared to bare CCY. Based on the high specific surface area of ZnO nanorods structure should be promising support materials for enzyme immobilization in sensor applications. Also, from the reversible redox reactions, the accessible surface area (A_e) value could be calculated using the standard Randle–Sevcik equation (Eq. 2.3). For this, we have maintained a uniform fiber length of 5 cm throughout the experiments. Approximately 4 cm length -fiber was soaked into the electrolyte solution. The calculated value of A_e is 0.0700 and 0.0932 cm^2 for bare CCY and ZnO NRs/CCY working electrode respectively. It could be speculated that only part of the total surface area of the electrode was accessible for the electron – transfer on the ZnO NRs/CCY working electrode.

5.3.7 Wettability analysis of CCY and ZnO NRs/CCY electrodes

In order to study the surface wettability behavior of the ZnO NRs array on CCY, the water contact angle (WCA) was evaluated and the outcome is shown in Fig. 5.9. Contact angle of a water droplet (2 mL) is used as the measure of wettability in this study. Each data point was averaged from five different Positions.

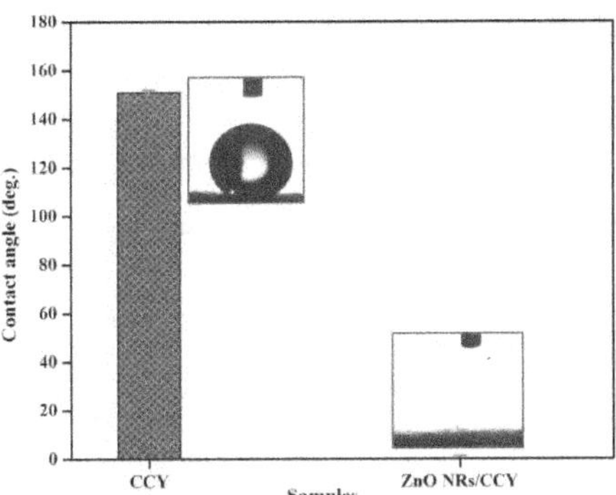

Fig. 5.9 Water contact angle of on CCY and ZnO NRs covered CCY [Insets: The images of water contact angle]

The bare CCY was found to be super hydrophobic, meaning the contact angle is larger than 150 °. After the coating of ZnO NRs array on carbon fabrics indicated a faster wetting time as the water droplet was absorbed immediately into the rods of the fabric. Water on this superhydrophilic ZnO NRs surfaces spread/ absorbed very quickly, and exhibited water contact angle close to zero. The insets showed the pictures of a water droplet with contact angle larger than 150° and close to zero states [50-52].

5.3.8 *In vitro* cell viability evaluation of CCY and ZnO NRs/CCY electrodes

Fig. 5.10 MTT analysis of cultured fibroblast L929 cells treated with different concentration of ZnO NRs on CCY samples for 24 hrs. Data represented as mean ± SD of three independent tests. **P<0.01

To analyze the biocompatibility of ZnO NRs/CCY (0.25, 0.5 and 1 mg/mL), we performed *in vitro* cell viability test using L929 cell line. The results showed good biocompatibility of the prepared ZnO NRs/CCY in concentration range of 0.25, 0.5 and 1 mg with the cell viability outcomes of 99.50, 99.25 and 98.84 respectively. Moreover, we did not notice any morphological defects after the incubation even for higher concentration of ZnO NRs/CCY (Fig. 5.10). This endorsed the biocompatibility nature of the ZnO NRs on CCY, It could act as a potential candidate in developing fiber based sensing platform which can be suitable for real time applications.

5.4 Electrochemical analysis

5.4.1 Cyclic voltammetry studies

The electrochemical behavior of the stepwise fabrication of immunosensor electrode was studied by CV technique. The CV curves on the bare CCY electrode, ZnO

NRs/CCY electrode, Anti-C$_{mab}$/ZnO NRs/CCY immunoelectrode and BSA/Anti-C$_{mab}$/ZnO NRs/CCY immunoelectrode were carried out in PBS (10 mM, pH 7.0) as shown in Fig. 5.10. The magnitude of the electrochemical current response for ZnO NRs/CCY electrode increased to ~268 µA. After the immobilization of Anti-C$_{mab}$ onto the ZnO NRs/CCY electrode, the electrochemical response current decreased to ~248 µA. This evidenced that successful binding of Anti-C$_{mab}$ with EDC/NHS-ZnO NRs/CCY immobilizing matrix further hindered the electrons passage from medium to electrode. Furthermore, the magnitude of current response further decreases (~232 µA) after the immobilization of BSA onto the Anti-C$_{mab}$/ZnO NRs/CCY immunoelectrode due to blocking of non-specific binding sites of Anti-C$_{mab}$ that insulate the electrode and perturb electron distribution.

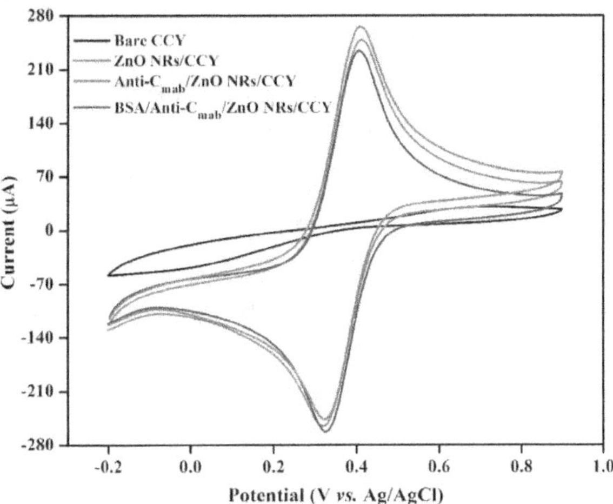

Fig. 5.10 CV analysis of step wise fabrication of BSA/Anti-C$_{mab}$/ZnO NRs/CCY immunoelectrode from CCY in PBS (10 mM, pH 7.0)

5.4.2 Effect of pH

The Fig. 5.11a shows the results of the BSA/Anti-C$_{mab}$/ZnO NRs/CCY immunoelectrode relating to the CV studies as a function of pH (4.5-8.5) in PBS. To prepare the immunosensor, it is necessary that the immobilized antibody should have retained its biological activity to bind with the antigen and this was found to be dependent on the immobilizing matrix and the pH of the working electrolyte.

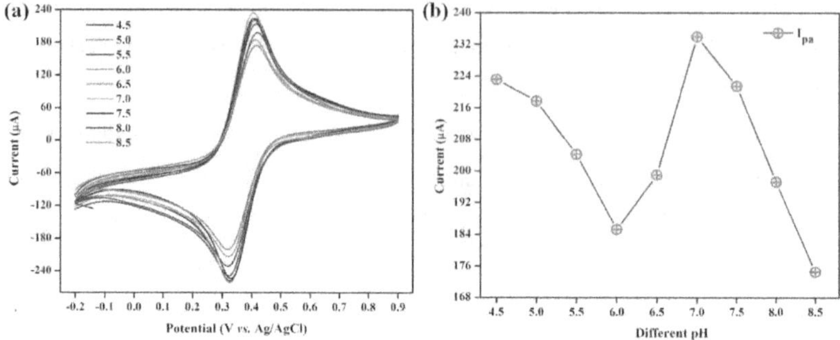

Fig. 5.11 (a) CV analysis of the BSA/Anti-C$_{mab}$/ZnO NRs/CCY immunoelectrode as a function of pH from 4.5 to 8.5 and (b) Linear plot of peak current *vs.* pH values

Thus, it is very key to optimize the pH of the immunoelectrode for the recognition of the analyte. It was observed that the magnitude of the oxidation and reduction peak response current vary of pH in the range of 4.5 to 8.5. However, most stable oxidation and reduction peak current response and highest peak current were observed for pH 7.0. Compared to other pH values and the linear plot of peak current *vs.* versus pH values was shown in Fig. 5.11b. Further increasing of pH, the oxidation peak current decreased. Hence, pH 7.0 was chosen which mimics biological environments and at this pH the electrode showed stable and repeatable response.

5.4.3 Effect of scan rate

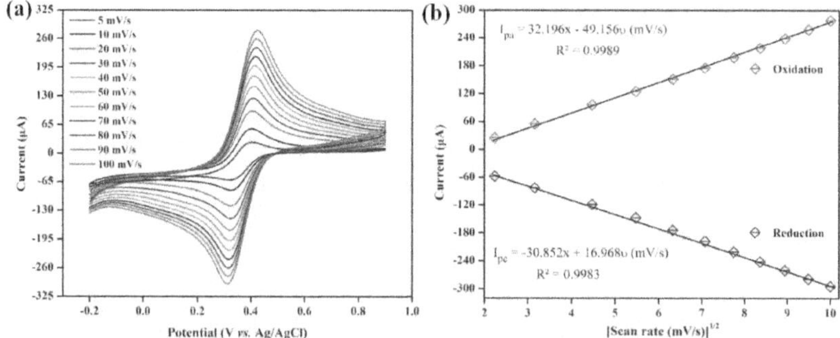

Fig. 5.12 (a) CV analysis of the BSA/Anti-C$_{mab}$/ZnO NRs/CCY immunoelectrode as a function of scan rates (5 to 100 mV/s) in PBS (10 mM, pH 7.0) and (b) Linear plot of the oxidation and reduction peak currents *vs.* square root of scan rates

The electrochemical performance of the prepared BSA/Anti-C$_{mab}$/ZnO NRs/CCY immunoelectrode has also been studied using CV studies as a function of scan rate from 5–100 mV/s (as shown in Fig. 5.12a).

The magnitude of the current response increased while increasing the scan rate. It is observed that the magnitude of the current response was linearly dependent (in Fig. 5.12b) on the scan rate and given in following equations (Eq. 5.8 & 5.9),

$$I_{pa}(\mu A) = 32.196x - 49.156\upsilon \ (mV/s); \ R^2 = 0.9989 \qquad ------(Eq.\,5.8)$$

$$I_{pc}(\mu A) = -30.852x + 16.968\upsilon \ (mV/s); \ R^2 = 0.9983 \qquad ------(Eq.\,5.9)$$

Well defined redox peaks suggested that the diffusion of the electrons was surface controlled electrochemistry. The stable redox peak current and position during repeated scans at a particular scan rate suggested that the prepared electrode exhibited a quasi-reversible process. It was observed that the immunoelectrode showed prominent redox peaks in PBS and exhibited stability up to 100 mV/s.

5.4.4 Cortisol response studies of BSA/Anti-C$_{mab}$/ZnO NRs/CCY immunoelectrode by CV

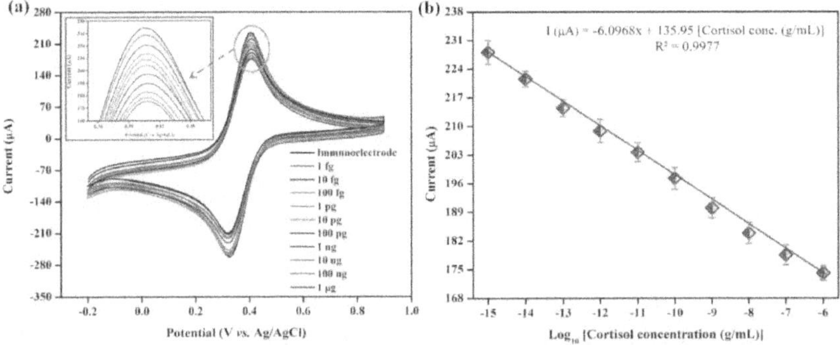

Fig. 5.13 (a) Electrochemical studies of BSA/Anti-C$_{mab}$/ZnO NRs/CCY immunoelectrode as a function of cortisol concentration varied from 1 fg to 1 µg in PBS (10 mM, pH 7.0) and (b) Linear plot between electrochemical peak current response and logarithm of cortisol concentration

The electrochemical response of the BSA/Anti-C_{mab}/ZnO NRs/CCY immunoelectrode has been studied as a function of cortisol concentration (Fig. 5.13) using CV technique in PBS (10 mM, pH 7.0). During the response study, the magnitude of the electrochemical response current of the BSA/Anti-C_{mab}/ZnO/CCY immunoelectrode was observed to decrease on increasing the cortisol concentration (Fig. 5.13a). This confirmed the successful formation of an immuno-complex between the cortisol and the Anti-cortisol antibody. The graph showing change in current with the log of concentration is almost linear and was expressed in following the equation (Eq. 5.10),

$$\Delta I\ (\mu A) = -6.0968x + 135.95\ [Cortisol\ conc.\ (g/mL);\ R^2 = 0.9977 - -(Eq.\,5.10)$$

A linear calibration curve (Fig. 5.13b) obtained between the logarithm of cortisol concentration and the magnitude of electrochemical current response showing good linear range from 1 fg - 1 μg, excellent response at low concentration of 1 fg/mL to upper limit of 1 μg/mL with a correlation coefficient of 0.9977. The detection limit of the fabricated immunosensor has been estimated as 0.45 fg.

5.4.5 Cortisol response studies of BSA/Anti-C_{mab}/ZnO NRs/CCY immunoelectrode by DPV

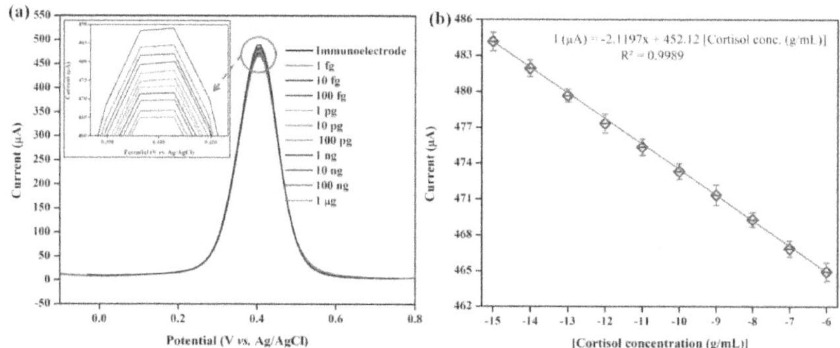

Fig. 5.14 (a) DPV analysis of the BSA/Anti-C_{mab}/ZnO NRs/CCY immunoelectrode as a function of cortisol concentration varied from 1 fg to 1 μg in PBS (10 mM, pH 7.0) and (b) Linear plot between electrochemical peak current response and logarithm of cortisol concentration

DPV studies of the BSA/Anti-C_{mab}/ZnO NRs/CCY immunoelectrode were carried out under similar condition used for CV. Fig. 5.14a revealed the insulating nature as decreasing peak current with increasing cortisol concentration. It is clear from Fig. 5.14b that with increasing cortisol concentration current decreased in the range of 1 fg to 1 µg, followed the linear equation (Eq. 5.11),

$$\Delta I \ (\mu A) = -2.1197x + 452.12 \ [Cortisol \ conc. \ (g/mL); \ R^2 = 0.9989 \ --(5.11)$$

The prepared immunoelectrode exhibited wide linear range of 1 fg to 1 µg with the lowest detection limit of 0.98 fg. This result confirmed from triplicate experiments have been done for each concentration on different electrodes that indicated by the error bars.

5.4.6 Interference studies

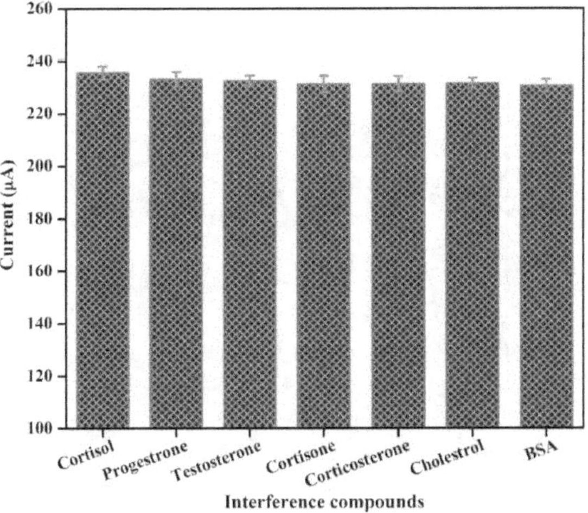

Fig. 5.15 Interference studies of BSA/Anti-C_{mab}/ ZnO NRs/CCY immunoelectrode towards Progesterone, Testosterone, Cortisone, Corticosterone, Cholesterol and BSA with respect to cortisol (100 ng/mL) in PBS (10 mM, pH 7.0)

The prepared BSA/Anti-C_{mab}/ZnO NRs/CCY immunoelectrode has been tested for interference compounds (100 ng/mL) such as **progesterone, testosterone, corticosterone, cortisone, cholesterol and BSA** with respect to cortisol have been studied using CV technique to check the specificity and selectivity (Fig. 5.15). This ZnO NRs based cortisol immunosensor exhibited significant electrochemical change only on adding cortisol and show minimum change on adding interferents (1–3%). The obtained results indicated that the fabricated BSA/Anti-C_{mab}/ZnO NRs/CCY immunoelectrodes were selective towards for cortisol.

5.4.7 Stability, repeatability and reproducibility studies

The CV studies related to the reproducibility of the BSA/Anti-C_{mab}/ZnO NRs/CCY immunosensors evidenced the consistent electrochemical response current up to 30 days after which retains the 96.23% after the storage at 4 °C, which indicated that the modified electrode has a long-term life time. Similarly, the stability of ZnO NRs/CCY immunoelectrode was examined by measuring the current response using cyclic voltammetry for 1000 cycles in 10 mM PBS as shown in Fig. 5.16. The RSD values were calculated from the current responses obtained for ZnO NRs/CCY of ±2 which demonstrating the good stability of the fiber.

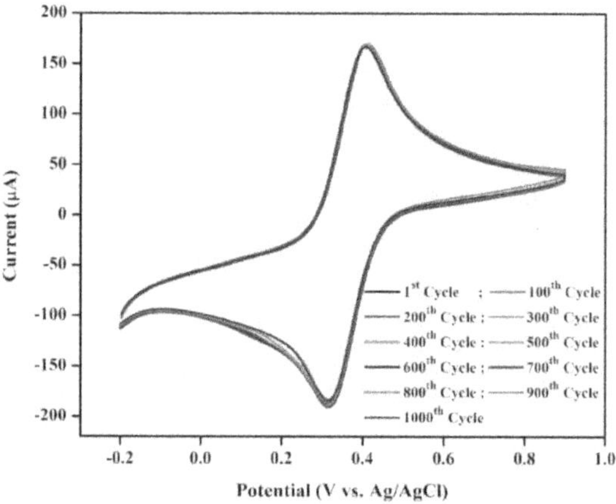

Fig. 5.16 The stability analysis of ZnO NRs/CCY immunoelectrode for 1000 cycles in 10 mM PBS

The RSD of 1.4% was found for 10 measurements of 100 ng/mL of cortisol by single BSA/Anti-C_{mab}/ZnO NRs/CCY immunoelectrode. The five BSA/Anti-C_{mab}/ZnO NRs/CCY immunoelectrode were prepared independently and applied for cortisol detection to appraise the reproducibility of the prepared electrode. The RSD of measurements was found as 2.8 % for cortisol, which was revealed the excellent reproducibility of binder free BSA/Anti-C_{mab}/ZnO NRs/CCY immunoelectrodes.

5.3.8 Real sample analysis

The fabricated cortisol immunosensor were used to detect human sweat cortisol and obtained results were validated using commercially CLIA sensing technique. This ZnO NRs based cortisol immunosensor were used for cortisol detection in human sweat collected at different time. The cortisol concentration of same sweat samples was detected using CILA and compared with the values measured using the prepared immunosensor. The results of both techniques are summarized in Table 5.1

Table 5.1 Comparison of sweat cortisol estimated using chemiluminescence immunoassay and ZnO/CCY based electrochemical immunosensor

Samples	CLIA method (ng/mL)	ZnO NRs/CCY immunosensor				
		Measured (ng/mL)*	Added (ng/mL)	Found (ng/mL)*	RSD (%)	Recovery (%)
1	24	22.54	50	75.03	4.46	99.02
2	27	24.87	50	73.34	2.33	97.95
3	54	53.25	50	101.67	3.13	98.46
4.	59	60.74	50	113.86	3.54	102.81
5.	71	68.56	50	132.88	3.84	103.36

*** The average value of three successive experiments.**

Herein, CV method was used to detect the cortisol level in sweat. The RSD of the proposed immunosensor from 2.33 % to 4.46 % and the recovery rates of the samples were ranged between 97.95 % and 103.36 %. The significant recovery percentages of cortisol in various sweat samples were determined. The outcome values were validated using commercially available CLIA sensing method and the results are shown in Fig. 5.17.

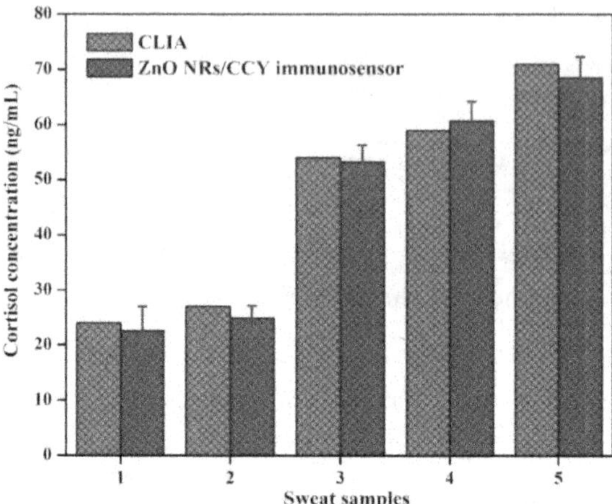

Fig. 5.17 Comparison graph of sweat cortisol estimated using chemiluminescence immunoassay and ZnO NRs/CCY based electrochemical immunosensor

5.4 Conclusions

In this chapter, we have prepared vertically aligned 1D ZnO NRs on CCY using hydrothermal method to prepare binder free, highly sensitive and selective electrochemical cortisol immunosensor. The ZnO NRs/CCY also exhibited notable physico-chemical properties which influenced its immunosensing performance and the resultant values were very closure to the Fe_2O_3/CCY immunoelectrode responses. However, we have incited to prepare carbon based electrodes to enhance the mechanical and conductive properties of the immunoelectrodes. Therefore, we analyzed the catalytic performance of MWCNTs integrated CCY towards cortisol sensing and the results were discussed in following chapter.

References

1. H. Ko, R. Kapadia, K. Takei, T. Takahashi, X. Zhang, A. Javey, Multifunctional, flexible electronic systems based on engineered nanostructured materials, *Nanotechnology,* **23** (2012) 344001 (1-11).

2. S. Wagner and S. Bauer, Materials for stretchable electronics, *MRS Bull.,* **37** (2012) 207-213.

3. K. Cherenack and L. V. Pieterson, Smart textiles: Challenges and opportunities, *J. Appl. Phys.,* **112** (2012) 091301 (1-14).

4. Y. Wu, H. Yan, M. Huang, B. Messer, J. H. Song, P. Yang, Inorganic semiconductor nanowires: rational growth, assembly and novel properties, *Chem. Eur. J.,* **8** (2002) 1260-1268.

5. M. Skompska and K. Zarebska, Electrodeposition of ZnO nanorod arrays on transparent conducting substrates–a review, *Electrochim. Acta,* **127** (2014) 467–488.

6. D. R. Lide, Hand Book of Chemistry and Physics, 71st edition, *Publisher : CRC, Boca Raton, FL* (1991) *ISBN: 10- 0849304717.*

7. P. K. Vabbina, A. Kaushik, N. Pokhrel, S. Bhansali, N. Pala, Electrochemical cortisol immunosensors based on sonochemically synthesized zinc oxide 1D nanorods and 2D nanoflakes, *Biosens Bioelectron.,* **63** (2015) 124–130.

8. S. Meng, Y. Hong, Z. Dai, W. Huang, X. Dong, Simultaneous detection of dihydroxybenzene isomers with ZnO Nanorod/Carbon cloth electrodes, *ACS Appl. Mater. Interfaces,* **9** (2017) 12453–12460.

9. X. Duan, Y. Huang, R. Agarwal, C. M. Lieber, Single-nanowire electrically driven lasers, *Nature,* **421** (2003) 241-245.

10. M. Law, D. J. Sirbuly, J. C. Johnson, J. Goldberger, R. J. Saykally, P. Yang, Nanoribbon waveguides for sub wavelength photonics integration, *Science,* **305** (2004) 1269-1273.

11. L. C. Tien, P. W. Sadik, D. P. Norton, L. F. Voss, S. J. Pearton, H. T. Wang, B. S. Kang, F. Ren, J. Jun, J. Lin, Hydrogen sensing at room temperature with Pt-coated ZnO thin films and nanorods, *Appl Phys Lett.,* **87** (2005) 222106 (1-3).

12. T. J. Hsueh , S. J. Chang, C. L. Hsu, Y. R. Lin, I. C. Chen, Highly sensitive ZnO nanowire ethanol sensor with Pd adsorption, *Appl Phys Lett.,* **91** (2007) 053111 (1-3).

13. V. Gupta and A. Mansingh, Influence of post deposition annealing on the structural and optical properties of sputtered zinc oxide film, *J Appl phys.,* **80** (1996) 1063–1073.

14. T. J. Athauda, P. Hari, R. R. Ozer, Tuning Physical and Optical Properties of ZnO Nanowire Arrays Grown on Cotton Fibers, *ACS Appl. Mater. Interfaces,* **5** (2013) 6237–6246.

15. S. Nozaki, S. Sarangi, K. Uchida and S. Sahu, Hydrothermal Growth of Zinc Oxide Nanorods and Glucose-Sensor Application, *Soft Nanosci. Lett,* **3** (2013) 23-32.

16. K. Khun, Z. H. Ibupoto, O. Nur, M. Willander, Development of Galactose biosensor based on functionalized ZnO Nanorods with Galactose Oxidase, *J. Sensors,* **696247** (2012) 1-7.

17. V. N. Psychoyios, G. P. Nikoleli, N. Tzamtzis, D. P. Nikolelis, N. Psaroudakis, B. Danielsson, M. Q. Israr, M. Willander, Potentiometric cholesterol biosensor based on ZnO nanowalls and stabilized polymerized lipid film, *Electroanalysis,* **25** (2013) 367 – 372.

18. X. C. Xiang, Y. Chi, Gu B. Xiang, F. S. Jiang, Nanostructured ZnO for biosensing applications, *Chin Sci Bull.,* **58** (2013) 58, 2563-2566.

19. C. Yang, B. Gu, D. Zhang, C. Gea, H. Tao, Coaxial Carbon Fiber/ZnO Nanorods as Electrodes for the Electrochemical Determination of Dopamine, *Anal. Methods,* **8** (2016) 650-655.

20. H. Chen,Y. Y. He, M. H. Lin, S. R. Lin, T. W. Chang, C. F. Lin, Chang, T. R. Y. Meng, L. Sheu, C. B. Chen, Y. S. Lin, Characterizations of zinc oxide nanorods incorporating a graphene layer as antibacterial nanocomposites on silicon substrates, *Ceram. Int.,* **42** (2016) 3424–3428.

21. M. H. Asif, S. M. U. Ali, O. Nur, M. Willander, C. Brannmark, P. Stralfors, U. H. Englund, F. Elinder, B. Danielsson, Functionalised ZnO-nanorod-based selective electrochemical sensor for intracellular glucose, *Biosens Bioelectron.,* **25** (2010) 2205–2211.

22. P. C. Chang, Z. Fan, D. Wang, W. Y. Tseng, W. A. Chiou, J. Hong, Jia G. Lu, ZnO Nanowires synthesized by vapor trapping CVD method, *Chem. Mater.,* **16** (2004) 5133-5137.

23. J. Zhou, N. Xu, Z. L. Wang, Dissolving behavior and stability of ZnO wires in biofluids: A Study on biodegradability and biocompatibility of ZnO nanostructures, *Adv. Mater.,* **18** (2006) 2432–2435.

24. Z. Li, R. Yang, M. Yu, F. Bai, C. Li, Z. L. Wang, Cellular level biocompatibility and biosafety of ZnO nanowires, *J. Phys. Chem. C,* **112** (2008) 20114-20117.

25. M.Q. Israr, J.R. Sadaf, M.H. Asif, O. Nur, M. Willander, B. Danielsson, Potentiometric cholesterol biosensor based on ZnO nanorods chemically grown on Ag wire, *Thin Solid Films,* **519** (2010) 1106–1109.

26. H.Liu, C. Gu, C. Hou, Z. Yin, K. Fan, M. Zhang, Plasma-assisted synthesis of carbon fibers/ZnO core–shell hybrids on carbon fiber templates for detection of ascorbic acid and uric acid, *Sens. Actuators, B-Chem,* **224** (2016) 857–862.

27. B. Tian and C. M. Lieber, Design, synthesis, and characterization of novel nanowire structures for photovoltaics and intracellular probes, *Pure Appl Chem.,* **83** (2011) 2153–2169.

28. Z. Zhao, W. Lei, X. Zhang, B. Wang, H. Jiang, ZnO-based amperometric enzyme biosensors, *Sensors,* **10** (2010) 1216–1231.

29. J. Wang, X. Sun, A. Wei, Y. Lei, X. Cai, C.M. Li, Z. N. Dong, Zinc oxide nanocombs biosensor for glucose detection, *Appl. Phys. Lett.,* **88** (2006) 233106 (1-3).

30. T. Kong, Y. Chen, Y. Ye, K. Zhang, Z. Wang, X. Wang, An amperometric glucose biosensor based on the immobilization of glucose oxidase on the ZnO nanotubes, *Sens. Actuators B-Chem,* **138** (2009) 344–350.

31. D. Pradhan, F. Niroui, K. Leung, High-performance, flexible enzymatic glucose biosensor based on ZnO nanowires supported on a gold-coated polyester substrate, *ACS Appl. Mater. Interfaces,* **2** (2010) 2409–2412.

32. R. D. Munje, S. Muthukumar, S. Prasad, Lancet-free and label-free diagnostics of glucose in sweat using Zinc Oxide based flexible bioelectronics, *Sens. and Actuators B-chem,* **238** (2017) 482–490.

33. S. P. Usha, A. M. Shrivastav, B. D. Gupta, A contemporary approach for design and characterization of fiberoptic-cortisol sensor tailoring LMR and ZnO/PPY molecularly imprinted film, *Biosens Bioelectron.*, **87** (2017) 178–186.

34. C. Yang, B. Gu, D. Zhang, C. Ge, H. Tao, Coaxial carbon fiber/ZnO nanorods as electrodes for the electrochemical determination of dopamine, *Anal. Methods,* **8** (2016) 650–655.

35. S. Meng, Y. Hong, Z. Dai, W. Huang, X. Dong, Simultaneous detection of dihydroxybenzene isomers with ZnO Nanorod/Carbon cloth electrodes, *ACS Appl. Mater. Interfaces,* **9** (2017) 12453−1246.0

36. A.Y. Boroujeni, M. A. Haik, A. Emami, R. Kalhor, Hybrid ZnO nanorod grafted carbon fiber reinforced polymer composites; randomly versus radially aligned long ZnO nanorods growth, *J. Nanosci. Nanotechnol.,* **18** (2017) 4182-4188.

37. M. H. Malakooti, H. S. Hwang, H. A. Sodano, Morphology-controlled ZnO nanowire arrays for tailored hybrid composites with high damping, *ACS Appl. Mater. Interfaces,* **7** (2015) 332-339.

38. Y. Bao, C. Wang, J. Ma, Morphology control of ZnO microstructures by varying hexamethylenetetramine and trisodium citrate concentration and their photocatalytic activity, *Mater. Des.,* **101** (2016) 7-15.

39. K.S. Ranjith, R.T. Rajendra Kumar, Surfactant free, simple, morphological and defect engineered ZnO nanocatalyst: Effective study on sunlight driven and reusable photocatalytic properties, *J. Photochem. Photobiol.,* **329** (2016) 35–45.

40. J. Cui, Defect control and its influence on the exciton emission of electrodeposited ZnO nanorods, *J. Phys. Chem. C,* **112** (2008) 10385–10388

41. P. Wang, D.Y. Liu, D.S. Li, Hydrothermal synthesis of different zinc oxide nanostructures: growth structure and gas sensing properties, *Mater. Trans.,* **53** (2012) 1892–1895.

42. D. Polsongkram, P. Chamninok, G. Chai, H. Khallaf, S. Pukird, S. Park, A. Schulte, Effect of synthesis conditions on the growth of ZnO nanorods via hydrothermal method, *Physica B,* **403** (2008) 3713–3717.

43. C. Liu, W. Zhang, J. Sun, J. Wen, Q. Yang, H. Cuo, X. Ma, M. Zhang, Piezoelectric nanogenerator based on a flexible carbon-fiber/ZnO–ZnSe bilayer structure wire, *Appl. Surf. Sci.*, **322** (2014) 95–100.

44. Shilpa, B. M. Basavaraja, S. B. Majumder, A. Sharma, Electrospun hollow glassy carbon–reduced graphene oxide nanofibers with encapsulated ZnO nanoparticles: a free standing anode for Li-ion batteries, *J. Mater. Chem. A*, **3** (2015) 5344-5351.

45. J. Fei, W. Luo, J. F. Huang, H. B. Ouyang, H. K. Wang, L, Y. Cao, Effect of hydrothermal modified carbon fiber through Diels–Alder reaction and its reinforced phenolic composites, *RSC Adv.*, **5** (2015) 64450–64455.

46. J. Song, Q. Yuan, X. Liu, D. Wang, F, Fu, W. Yang, Combination of nitrogen plasma modification and waterborne polyurethane treatment of carbon fiber paper used for electric heating of wood floors, *BioResources*, **10** (2015) 5820-5829.

47. J. Fei, D. Luo, J. Huang, C. Zhang, X. Duan, L. Zhang, Growth of aligned ZnO nanorods on carbon fabric and its composite for superior mechanical and tribological performance, *Surf. Coat. Technol.*, **344** (2018) 433-440.

48. R. Cuscó, E. A. Lladó, J. Ibáñez, L. Artús, Temperature dependence of Raman scattering in ZnO, *Phy. Rev B*, **75** (2007) 165202 (1-11).

49. X. Liu, H. Du, X. W. Sun, B. Liu, D. Zhao, H. Sun, Visible-light photoresponse in a hollow microtube–nanowire structure made of carbon-doped ZnO, *CrystEngComm*, **14** (2012) 2886–2890.

50. M. Lee, G. Kwak, K. Yong, Wettability control of ZnO nanoparticles for universal applications, *ACS Appl. Mater. Interfaces*, **3**, (2011) 3350–3356.

51. K. S. Ranjith, R. Pandian, E. McGlynn, R. T. Rajendra Kumar, Alignment, morphology and defect control of vertically aligned ZnO nanorod array: Competition between "Surfactant" and "Stabilizer" roles of the amine species and its photocatalytic properties, *Cryst. Growth Des.*, **14** (2014) 2873−2879.

52. L. He, A. Karumuri, S. M. Mukhopadhyay, Wettability tailoring of nanotube carpets: morphology-chemistry synergy for hydrophobic– hydrophilic cycling, *RSC Adv.*, **7** (2017) 25265–25275.

Chapter VI

Estimation of Stress Biomarker Using Dip Coated MWCNTs on Conductive Yarn in Human Sweat

Highlights

- ❧ Multiwall carbon nanotubes (MWCNTs) were integrated on CCY by a traditional dip-coating process.

- ❧ The coating time greatly influenced the electrical performance of MWCNTs/CCY hybrids.

- ❧ The optimized MWCNTs coating on CCY directly used as binder free immunoelectrode in cortisol estimation.

- ❧ The wide linear detection range and lower detection limit ensured the sensing ability of MWCNTs immunoelectrode.

- ❧ The prepared immunoelectrode can be used as functional materials for wearable electronics and smart textiles

Graphical illustration of immobilization and electrochemical immunosensing of cortisol on dip coated MWCNTs/CCY with possible redox mechanism

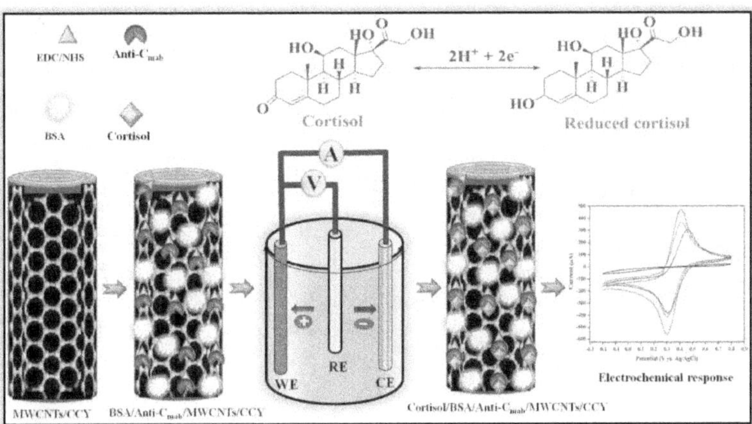

6.1 Introduction

A carbon nanotube (CNT) is one of the carbon allotropes such as graphite, graphene, diamond, fullerene and amorphous carbon. But, it is the one-dimensional carbon form which can have an aspect ratio greater than 1000 makes it interesting. The bonding in CNTs is sp^2, with each atom joined to three neighbors, as in graphite. CNTs are rolled-up graphene sheets (graphene is an individual graphite layer). This type of structural bonding, which is stronger than the sp^3 bonds found in diamond, provides unique strength to the molecules. Under high pressure, CNTs can merge together, trading some sp^2 bonds for sp^3 bonds having the possibility to form lengthy wires through high pressure nanotube linking [1, 2]. These carbon-based materials have high electrical conductivity, superior mechanical properties, light weight, flexibility and large aspect ratio [3-7]. Because of these unique features, the carbon materials are used in a wide range of fields, including energy storage, biology and medicine [8]. However, despite the abundant advantages, researcher still face challenges regarding the complex synthesis strategies, lack in uniformity and reproducibility of carbon materials. To overcome these issues and develop new applications of these materials with specific and precise properties is primordial [9].

CNTs were discovered by *Sumio lijima* (Japan) in 1991, which opened up a new area in field of material science and it is a minor by product of fullerene synthesis [10]. A CNT is a tube-shaped material, made up of carbon, having a diameter in nanometer scale, while length-to-diameter ratio of up to 132,000,000:1. CNTs have many forms of structures, thickness, length and number of layers. Outstanding progress has been made in the ensuring last few decades including the discovery of two basic types as single and multiwall carbon nanotubes [11].

6.1.1 Types of CNTs

The CNTs are of two types namely:

- φ Single walled carbon nanotubes (SWCNTs)

- φ Multiple walled carbon nanotubes (MWCNTs)

6.1.2 Single walled carbon nanotubes (SWCNTs)

SWCNTs consist of a single cylindrical carbon layer with a diameter of 0.4 - 2 nm, depending on the temperature at which they have been synthesized. It was found that the higher growth temperature yield larger the diameter of CNTs [12] as shown in Fig. 6.1. The structure of SWCNTs may be armchair, zigzag, chiral, or helical arrangements [13]. The SWCNTs have an ultrahigh surface area as large as 1300 m^2/g, which provide sufficient space for drug loading and bio conjugation [14]. SWCNT consists of two separate regions with different physical and chemical properties. The first is the sidewall of the tube and the second is the end cap of the tube. SWCNTs are one of the important varieties of CNTs because they exhibit important electric properties that are not shared by the MWCNT variants. The most basic building block of these systems is the electric wire therefore SWCNTs can be served as excellent conductors. SWCNTs are still very expensive to produce and the development of more inexpensive synthesis techniques is crucial to the future of carbon nanotechnology.

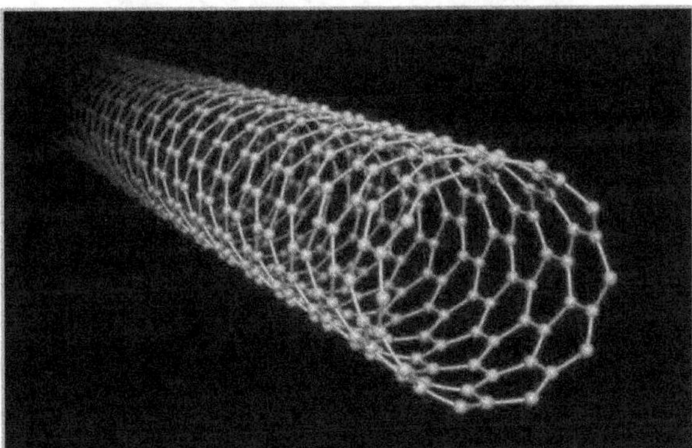

Fig. 6.1 Structure of single-walled carbon nanotubes

6.1.3 Multi-walled carbon nanotubes (MWCNTs)

MWCNTs consist of several coaxial cylinders, each made of a single graphene sheet surrounding a hollow core. The outer diameter of MWCNTs ranges from 2-100 nm, while the inner diameter is in the range of 1-3 nm and their length is in the order of one to several micrometers [15]. The sp^2 hybridization in MWCNTs, a delocalized electron cloud around the wall is generated is responsible for the interactions between adjacent cylindrical layers in MWCNTs resulting in a less flexible and more structural defects [16]. MWCNTs structures can be split into two categories based on their arrangements of graphite layers: one has a Parchment model which consists of a graphene sheet rolled up around it and the other is known as the Russian doll model where layers of graphene sheets are arranged within a concentric structure as shown in Fig. 6.2 [17].

Decoration of MWCNTs consists of depositing nanoparticles on their walls or ends, bonded by physical interaction with potential applications in catalysis, biosensors, biomedical, magnetic data storage and electronic devices. The various methods used for the synthesis of MWCNTs based hybrids include precipitation, hydrolysis at high temperature or chemical decomposition of a metal precursor [18, 19].

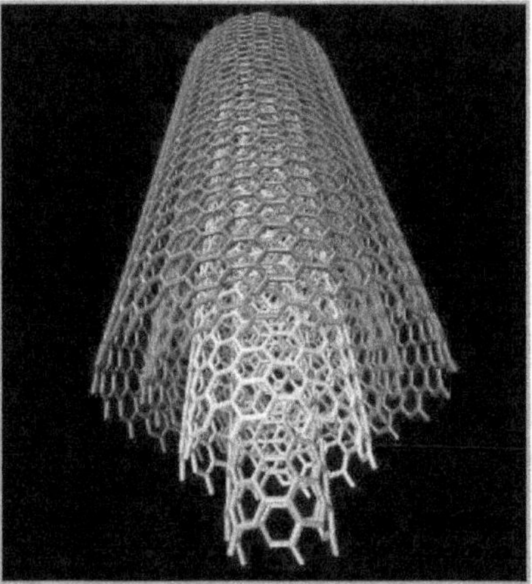

Fig. 6.2 Structure of multi-walled carbon nanotubes

6.1.4 Synthesis of CNTs

CNTs are generally produced by three main techniques: arc discharge, laser ablation and chemical vapor deposition (Shown in Fig. 6.3).

In arc discharge technique, a vapor is created by an arc discharge between two carbon electrodes with or without catalyst. The self-assembled CNTs will be formed from the resulting carbon vapor. In the laser ablation technique, a high power laser beam impinges on a volume of carbon containing feedstock gas (such as methane or carbon monoxide). Laser ablation was the first technique used to generate fullerenes in clusters. In this process, a piece of graphite is vaporized by laser irradiation under an inert atmosphere. This results in soot containing CNTs which are cooled at the walls of a quartz tube [20, 21]. At the moment, laser ablation produces a small amount of clean CNTs, whereas arc discharge methods generally produce large quantities of CNTs with impurities.

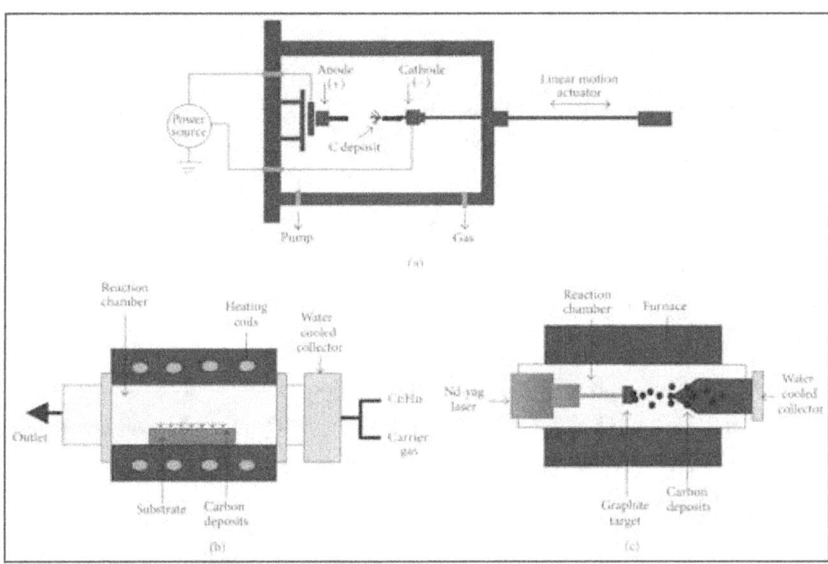

Fig. 6.3 Schematic illustration of methods used for CNTs synthesis (a) arc discharge, (b) CVD and (c) laser ablation

The CVD has exposed the most promise technique in terms of its price/unit ratio due to outstanding heat and mass transfer ensuing a homogeneous product, inherent scalability and comparatively low cost [22, 23]. CVD generally involves reacting a carbon containing gas (such as acetylene, ethylene and ethanol) with a metal catalyst particle (usually nickel, cobalt, iron or a mixture of these such as cobalt/iron or cobalt/molybdenum) at temperatures above 600 °C [24 , 25].

B. S. Shim *et al.*, demonstrated a simple process of transforming general commodity cotton threads into intelligent e-textiles using a polyelectrolyte-based CNTs via dip coating method. Efficient charge transport through the CNTs network (20 Ω/cm), improved their mechanical properties and the possibility to engineer tunneling junctions make them promising materials for many high-knowledge-content garments along with integrated humidity sensing. Also, CNT-cotton yarn used to detect albumin (the key protein of blood) with high sensitivity and selectivity. They suggested that the proof-of-concept provide a direct pathway for the application of these materials as wearable bio-monitoring and telemedicine sensors which are simple, sensitive, selective and versatile functional materials for wearable electronics and smart textiles [26].

Sharma *et al.,* reported that the CNTs were directly grown on carbon fiber (CFs) substrate by catalytic decomposition of acetylene precursor using thermal CVD process. The composites made of CNTs coated CFs showed 69 % higher tensile strength as compared to the composites made from carbon fiber which had undergone other heat treatment but without CNTs growth. They suggested that the application of CNTs grown CFs as reinforcement in other materials matrix could result in composites with enhanced tensile strength [27]. Also, E. T. Thostenson *et al.,* explained the synthesis of CNTs on the surface of CFs and the fiber/matrix interfacial properties were assessed using the single-fiber fragmentation test. They found that the presence of CNTs at the fiber/matrix interface improves the interfacial shear strength of the composites [28].

Wu (2016) *et al.,* constructed an integrated 3D CNTs forest/CC electrode for Li–polysulfide battery applications. They achieved high specific capacities of ~1200 mA h g^{-1} and ~800 mA h g^{-1} at 0.1 C and 1 C, respectively. They also found that the specific capacity was retained as 623 mA h g^{-1} after 300 cycles at 0.5 C [29]. Wang *et al.,* successfully developed a graphene oxide assisted a porous hybrid G–CNTs layer on the surface of CC. They concluded that the as-prepared G–CNT/CC was used as advanced binder-free electrodes for flexible supercapacitors, which showed significantly enhanced supercapacitor performance in terms of specific capacitance, rate capability, energy and power density due to the development of porous structure and enhanced conductivity facilitated by CNTs [30].

Barsan *et al.,* reported CNTs and nitrogen doped CNTs modified CC materials were employed for the first time in the development of new electrode sensor materials which were characterized by CV and EIS. The voltammetric response of model electroactive species showed a close to reversible electrochemical behavior, under diffusion control for functionalized electrodes. The immobilization of GOx on the both the electrodes lead to very robust biosensors that exhibited the highest sensitivity and LOD, underlying again the importance of CNT doping. Also, these electrodes indicated good stability, retaining enzyme activity and the possibility of dry storage brings further benefits, as it hinder enzyme leaching [31].

Wang *et al.,* developed a multifunctional, wearable, fabric sensor for monitoring small human motions, as well as vitals such as respiration rate and body temperature. The fabric sensors leveraged the mechanical and electrical properties of MWCNTs based nanocomposites. The results showed that they exhibited stable and repeatable strain sensing properties and strain sensitivity increased as higher concentrations of MWCNTs. Finally they suggested that these MWCNT-based fabric sensors could potentially be used for applications such as multifunctional wearable sensors or be integrated as part of 'smart garments' [32].

Regarding our work Tlili *et al.,* described the development and proof-of-concept testing of an ultrasensitive, label-free immunosensor based on chemiresistive transducer for cortisol detection using SWCNTs. The immunosensor demonstrated LOD of 1 pg/mL and excellent binding selectivity for cortisol even in the presence of structurally similar cortisol analagues such as 21-hydroprogesterone [33]. In 2013, A novel nanocomposite electrode material constituted of gold nanoparticles (AuNPs), MWCNTs n-octylpyridinium hexafluorophosphate (OPPF6) ionic liquid was prepared and checked for the development of electrochemical cortisol sensing devices by Guzmán group [34]. The prepared AuNPs/MWCNTs/OPPF$_6$ paste electrodes exhibited linear detection range of 0.1 - 10 ng/mL with a detection limit of 15 pg/mL. Also, the developed biosensor was applied to the analysis of human serum for real sample analysis.

Recently our collaborative group Manickam *et al.,* fabricated the electrochemical cortisol sensor using metalloporphyrin (MTPP) and the MWCNTs on screen printed carbon electrodes (SPCE). The cortisol sensor exhibited within the linear range of 50 fM to 100 nM with lowest limit of detection as 50 fM. The proposed screen printed cortisol sensor was used to accurately detect variations in salivary cortisol levels in young adult women and the accuracy of the sensor was validated with commercial ELISA assay and found to be correlated [35].

In this *Chapter VI*, we have reported that the catalytic activity of MWCNTs integrated CCY in the sweat cortisol detection. This MWCNTs/CCY immunoelectrode was directly used as the binder free working electrode for electrochemical detection of cortisol. The combination of CCY with MWCNTs was found to be sensitive to cortisol redox reaction due to their active catalytic sites and enhanced electrochemical activity. The prepared immunosensor was found to have wide linear range (10 fg – 1 µg) and a detection limit as low as 0.5 fg/mL. The sensor was further evaluated using human sweat samples, which demonstrating an accurate and reproducible platform for rapid detection of cortisol and validated with commercially available CILA method.

6.2. Materials and methods

6.2.1 Chemicals and reagents

Commercially available MWCNTs having an average diameter of 9.5 nm and length of 1.5 µm were used as starting materials, nitric acid (HNO_3), sulfuric acid (H_2SO_4), Dimethyl formamide (DMF) was purchased from Sigma Aldrich. All the chemicals were of analytical grade and used as received and DD water was used throughout the experiment.

6.2.2 MWCNTs functionalization

The surface treatment of MWCNTs with acid, oxidizing agents and surfactants produce carboxylic, hydroxyl and ketonic groups which alter the properties like dispersion stability and better interactions with the textile matrix. It is expected that these functional groups on the MWCNTs will interact with the carbon fiber matrix. Hydrogen bonding between the materials leads to the favorable MWCNTs-CCY interfacial bonding [36]. The functionalization of MWCNTs was carried out in a round-bottomed flask equipped with a reflux condenser and a thermometer [37]. Before the oxidation process, 200 mg of raw MWCNTs were taken in the mixture of concentrated HNO_3 and H_2SO_4 (200 mL) in the ratio of 1:3 at room temperature (28 ± 1 °C). The mixture was kept under ultrasonication for 3 hrs and poured into the refluxing round bottomed flask at 110 °C for 6 hrs. The acid solution reached room temperature it was filtered through a polytetrafluoroethylene membrane. The filtered substance was washed repeatedly with DD water till the filtrate was reached neutral. The final product was dried in a vacuum oven at 60 °C for 48 hrs.

6.2.3 Dip coating of MWCNTs on CCY

Generally, MWCNTs used to disperse in organic solvents like dichloro-methane, ethanol, isopropyl alcohol and THF etc. But in these solvents, MWCNTs have generally poor dispersion because of the high aspect ratio and poor van der Waal's interaction. In our work, we have chosen DMF because it is an aprotic solvent whose dielectric constant is 7.6. It is used as a moderate polar solvent and can dissolve a wide range of non-polar and polar chemical compounds with low evaporation rate. DMF is also reported as effective for separating and suspending CNTs. In the present work, the MWCNTs were dispersed in DMF in the ratio of 1:1 [38, 39].

Dipping method for modifying fabric is the most convenient approach used in the processing of fabric and should be considered to have great advantage over other methods due to its simplicity and the ability to integrate with existing processing steps.

The dispersed MWCNTs were coated on CCY surface with the regular dipping time intervals as 5,10,15,20, 25 and 30 seconds. The resulting MWCNTs coated yarns were collected and rinsed with alcohol and DD water three times to remove the loosely attached products or residues on their surfaces. Finally, the coated yarns were dried at 60 °C overnight and the conductivity of the coated yarns at different dipping time intervals were measured. To check the loading capacity of MWCNTs on CCY, the mass of fabric was measured before and after the dip coating. A uniform fiber length of 5 cm was used throughout the experiments.

6.2.4 Immobilization of Anti-C_{mab} onto MWCNTs/CCY

Covalent immobilization of Anti-C_{mab} on MWCNTs/CCY was achieved using EDC as the coupling agent and NHS as the activator. For binding 120 µl of 2 µg/mL Anti-C_{mab} solution in PBS (10 mM, pH 7) containing 0.4 M of EDC and NHS was poured onto the MWCNTs/CCY electrode and incubated for 120 mins in a humid chamber. The fabricated Anti-C_{mab}/MWCNTs/CCY electrode was washed with PBS, followed by 30 mins of incubation in 80 μL of 10 μg/mL BSA solutions in PBS for blocking of non-specific binding sites. The fabricated BSA/Anti-C_{mab}/MWCNTs/CCY immunoelectrode was washed several times and stored at 4 °C when not in use. And finally the BSA/Anti-C_{mab}/MWCNTs/CCY immunoelectrodes were analyzed for further electrochemical studies.

6.3 Results and discussion

6.3.1 XRD analysis of CCY and MWCNTs/CCY

Figure 6.4 compares the XRD patterns of bare CCY and MWCNTs coated CCY. It was evident from Fig. 6.4, the pattern showed a broad diffraction peak at ~26° that can be indexed to the (002) plane of pure carbon yarn. The other characteristic diffraction peaks of carbon were observed around 43.4° and 53.2° associated with (100) and (004) diffraction planes of graphite, respectively [40]. The relative sharpness of the peak of MWCNTs on CCY further confirmed that the graphitic structure of MWCNTs was preserved even after the dip coating. This protocol regulated the uniform coating without significantly damaging or degrading the overall crystallinity of the MWCNTs [31, 41].

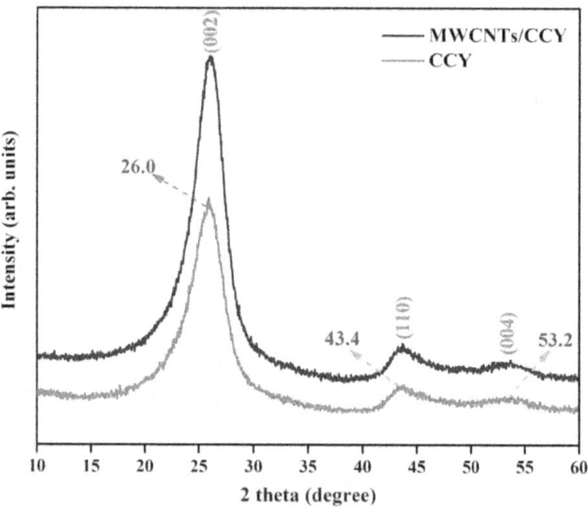

Fig. 6.4 X-ray diffraction patterns of CCY and MWCNTs/CCY

6.3.2 FT-IR spectra of CCY and MWCNTs/CCY

The dip coating of MWCNTs onto the CCY was further investigated by FT-IR spectra as shown in Fig. 6.5. The IR spectra of CCY shows a strong absorption band at 3410 cm^{-1} corresponds to O-H stretching vibration due to small amounts of absorbed water. A characteristic peak at 1586 cm^{-1} corresponds to C=C bond. The stretching vibration peak at 1037 cm^{-1} is assigned to C-O-C bond and the peak at 1734 cm^{-1} corresponds to C=O group of carbon in the CCY [42]. The absorption peaks at 2919 and 2852 cm^{-1} are due to C=H stretching. The high intensity peaks of asymmetric and symmetric stretching of C-H bonds are observed at 2923 and 2850 cm^{-1}, respectively. The stretching of C=O of the group is observed at 1751 cm^{-1} for MWCNTs which shifted towards higher energy compared to CCY (1734 cm^{-1}). Also, The stretching of C=C, O-H bending deformation in -COOH and C-O bond stretching in the MWCNTs are observed at 1639, 1452 and 1067 cm^{-1} indicating that carboxyl and hydroxyl groups were attached to the surface of MWCNTs. The results exhibited that the successful and uniform coating of MWCNTs on CCY [43, 44].

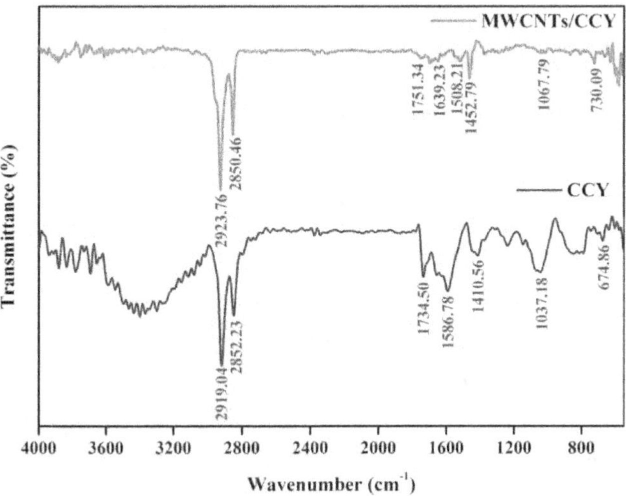

Fig. 6.5 FT-IR spectra of CCY and MWCNTs/CCY

6.3.3 Raman spectra of CCY and MWCNTs/CCY

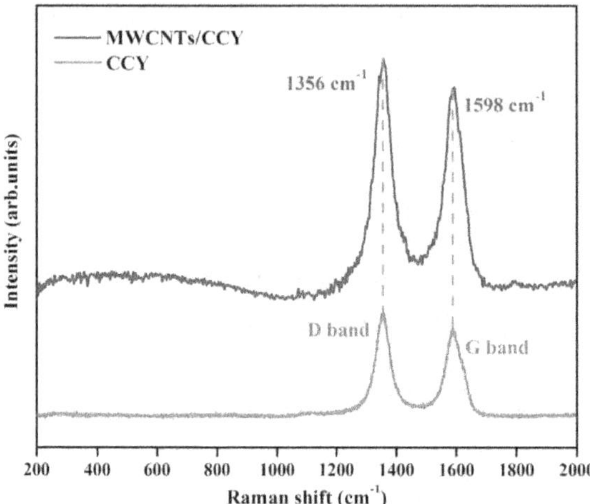

Fig. 6.6 Raman spectra of CCY and MWCNTs/CCY

In the Fig. 6.6, The broad characteristic peaks around 1356 and 1598 cm^{-1} were observed due to the D band (disordered carbon) and G band (graphitic carbon), respectively. The D-band corresponds to the disordered or sp^3-hybridized carbons in the MWCNTs wall and the G-band is assigned to vibrations of sp^2-bonded carbon atoms in graphene-like structures. The intensity ratio of D and G bands (I_D/I_G) was determined for CCY as 1.19 which designated the carbon fibers has been partially graphitized [45, 46]. The intensity ratio of the D and G bands i.e. (I_D/I_G ratio) helps to estimate the defects of carbon based samples where a higher ratio ensures more defects on carbon. The calculated I_D/I_G ratio for MWCNTs/CCY was 1.15, which was slightly varied from CCY due to some defect presence at sidewall of MWCNTs after oxidation process. No peaks shifts were observed in the graphitic peaks except their intensity values in MWCNTs after the 15 sec dip coating with CCY matrix [47]. This result ensured that the oxidation agents haven't destroyed the graphitic structure of MWCNTs.

6.3.4 Morphological and compositional analysis of CCY and MWCNTs/CCY

Figure 6.7a shows the morphology of pure CCY which consists of smaller fibers with smooth surface. The Fig. 6.7b shows the clearer picture of the smooth fiber in close magnification. The as-prepared and optimized MWCNTs (15 sec dipped) integrated onto CCY at were illustrated in different magnifications (Fig. 6.7 (c-f)). The FESEM images showed that the presence of MWCNTs homogenously covered the entire surface of CCY because the dip coating, a convenient coating method [48]. The interconnected construction of MWCNTs significantly improved the electrolyte-accessible surface area and consequently enhances its electrochemical activity towards cortisol.

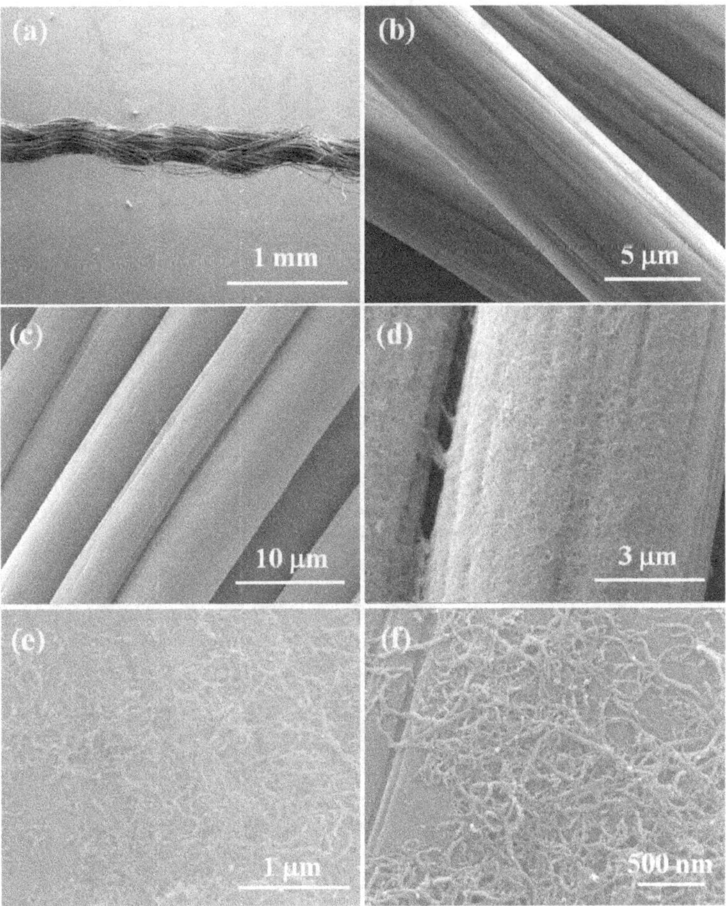

Fig. 6.7 FESEM images of (a, b) bare CCY and (c-f) MWCNTs/CCY with different magnifications

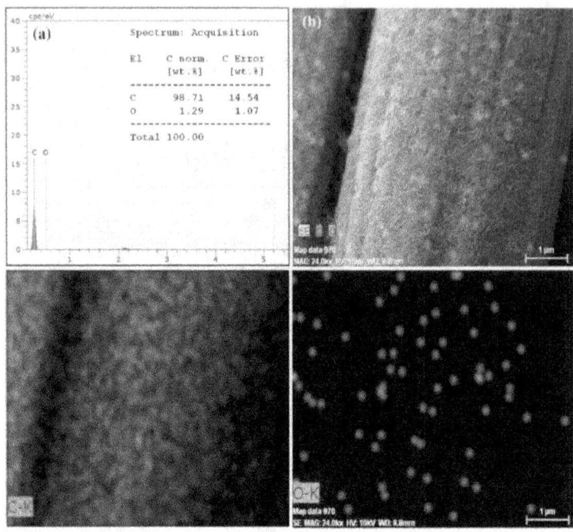

Fig. 6.8 (a) EDS spectra and (b) EDS mapping of MWCNTs/CCY

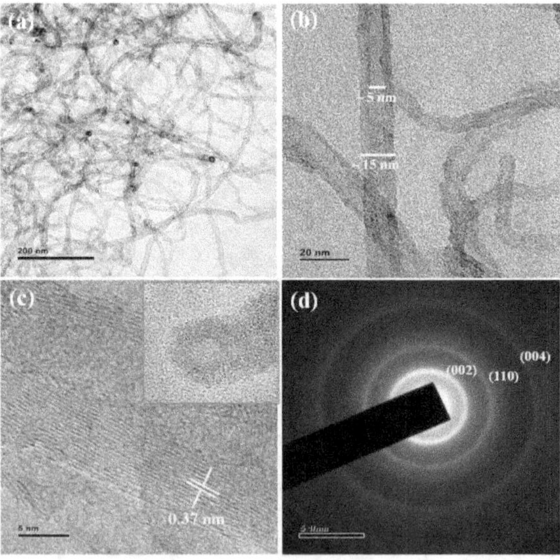

Fig. 6.9 (a) TEM image (b,c) HRTEM images and (d) SAED pattern of MWCNTs [inset: center of MWCNTs]

The EDS study was also performed for the chemical analysis of the MWCNTs integrated fibers and the results are given in Fig. 6.8a. The EDS spectra showed the peaks corresponding to C (99.38 wt. %), O (0.83 wt. %) as given in inset table. The absence of possible residues confirmed that the purity of integrated of MWCNTs on the CCY. The chemical composition further confirmed from EDS mapping (Fig. 6.8b) further evidenced the distribution of C and O elements on the surface CCY.

HRTEM imaging is used to measure the actual diameter and interlayer spacing of the MWCNTs. Fig. 6.9 shows characteristic HRTEM images of oxidized MWCNTs with different magnifications after the dispersion on a Cu grid. It showed the the diameter of MWCNTs studied including the high resolution lattice image. The HRTEM image in Fig. 6.9c also suggested the oxidized MWCNTs to be consisting of concentrically nested ~16 graphene sheets with the outer and inner diameters of ~15 and ~ 5 nm, respectively (Fig. 6.9 b&c). The interlayer distance was around 0.37 nm which accordance with the XRD results. Also, the inset (Fig. 6.9c) showed the the center of MWCNTs. The SAED pattern showed the concentric rings which indicated the amorphous nature of the material (Fig. 6.9d).

6.3.5 Electrical conductivity and mechanical properties of CCY and MWCNTs/CCY

Carbon-based materials such as carbon fiber, MWCNTs, SWCNTs and chemically modified graphite and graphene have been used either as conductive filler for composites or as base materials for films because of their high electrical conductivity. Well dispersed MWCNTs possess higher electrical conductivity than SWCNTs [49]. Figure 6.10a represent the electrical conductivity of MWCNTs/CCY were prepared with different dip coating (5-30 sec) cycles. The coating process significantly affected the electrical conductivity of the prepared MWCNTs/CCY with respect of dipping time. The prepared MWCNTs/CCY composites showed higher electrical conductivity of 27.78 S cm^{-1} for 15 sec dip coated yarn whereas bare CCY exhibited the conductivity of 5 S cm^{-1}.

The conductivity of the MWCNTs/CCY composites increased while increasing the dipping time and reached the maximum of 27.78 S cm^{-1} for 15 sec. Further increased the dipping time up to 30 sec, the conductivity gradually decreased. The reduction of the conductivity occurred probably due to the interface resistance and the resistance due to the elevation of the thickness of MWCNTs on CCY. The fairly low electrical resistance of MWCNTs coated yarn allows for convenient sensing applications that may not require any additional electronic supports or converters [28]. Also, conductivity of MWCNTs/CCY (15 sec) was demonstrated by powering an LED device connected to a battery as shown in Fig. 6.10b.

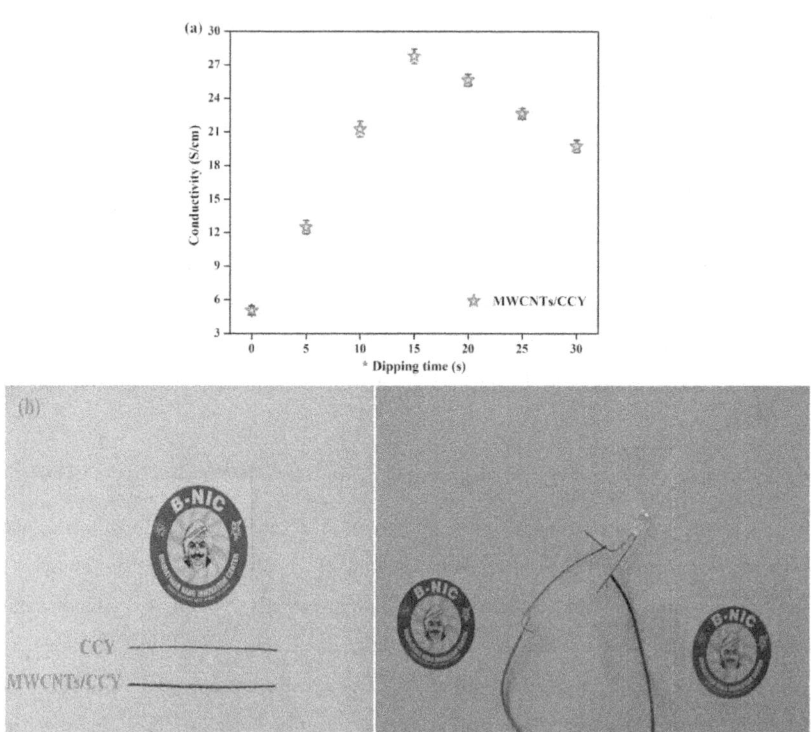

Fig. 6.10 (a) Electrical conductivity measurement of MWCNTs/CCY as function of dipping time and (b) Demonstration of LED emission with the current passing through MWCNTs/CCY

The strength of the MWCNTs coated CCY is more than 2 times higher than that of the uncoated yarn thread due to a reduction of the overall diameter, densification and stronger adhesion of the fibers to each other by the MWCNTs. The mechanical properties of the bare and MWCNTs coated CCY were analyzed and the ultimate strength was found as 20.10 MPa and 40.82 MPa along with the young modulus values of 37.17 and 82.74 MPa respectively. The higher young's modulus value of MWCNTs on CCY is highly preferred for the wearable sensor applications. The breaking strain (0.48 and 0.38) and elongation (5.27 and 7.53 %) were corresponding to CCY and MWCNTs/CCY.

6.3.6 Specific and assessable surface area of CCY and MWCNTs/CCY electrode

The specific surface areas were calculated using BET surface analysis for the CCY and MWCNTs/CCY and the values were determined as 75.60 m^2/g and 122.54 m^2/g. Clearly, network like interconnected MWCNTS on CCY possessed higher specific surface area as compared to bare CCY.

The electrochemically active surface area of electrodes was examined by using the stranded Randles-Sevcik equation (Eq. 2.3). The calculated electrochemically active surface area is 0.0734 and 0.0858 cm^2 for the bare CCY and MWCNTs coated CCY respectively.

6.3.7 Wettability analysis of CCY and MWCNTs/CCY electrodes

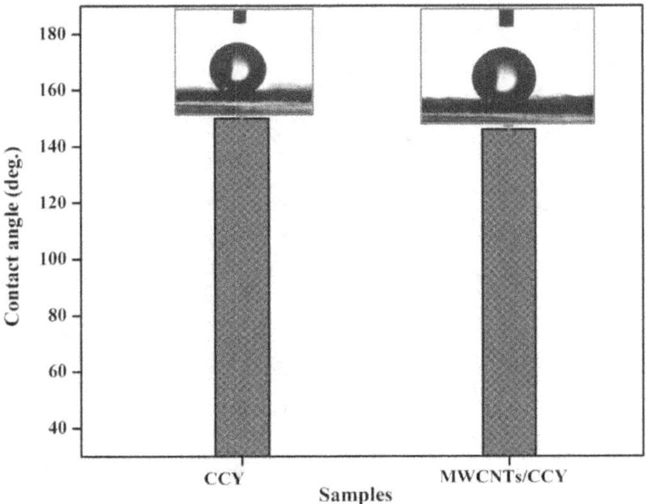

Fig. 6.11 Water contact angle of on CCY and MWCNTs modified CCY [Insets: The images of water contact angle]

Wettability was tested across physiologically stiff and soft accommodating CCY substrates and it was shown in Fig. 6.11 to be hydrophobic before dip coating of MWCNTs. After the coating of MWCNTs on CCY, the contact angle value was observed as 150° which might be attributed from hydrophobic surface of randomly arranged and interconnected MWCNTs [50]. The densed and uniform coating of MWCNTs was used to stabilize the super-hydrophobicity through Salvinia effect. As it occurs in Salvinia, water droplets are pinned by the attractive interaction due to hydrophilic carbonaceous nanostructures, while they exhibited super-hydrophobic contact angles with a huge amount of air pockets, owing to the repulsive interaction of hydrophobic MWCNTs [51, 52].

6.4 Electrochemical analysis

6.4.1. CV response for MWCNTs/CCY as function of dipping time

The Figure 6.12 represents the CV response of MWCNTs coated CCY as function of dipping time. The time interval was set as 5-30 sec in 5 sec interval. The redox peaks were found to be increased upto 15 sec dipping time. Further increasing the dipping time the redox peak current found to be gradually decreased. It's due to the interfacial resistance and elevation of the thickness of MWCNTs onto CCY. This result is very well matched with the electrical conductivity results (Fig. 6.10a).

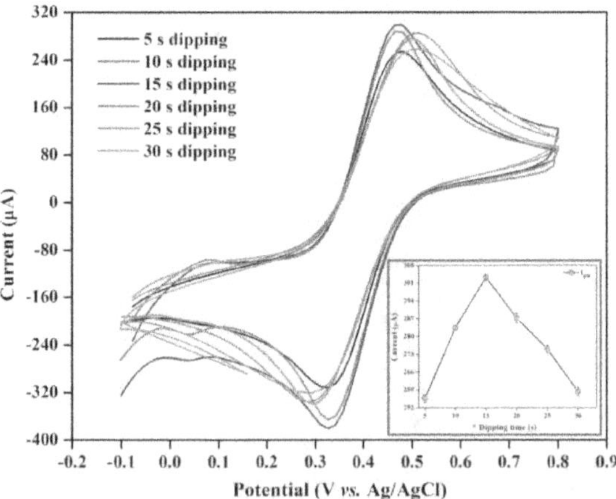

Fig. 6.12 CV response of MWCNTs/CCY as function of dipping time [Inset: Dipping time vs. Current response]

6.4.2 Cyclic voltammetry studies

Bare CCY electrode (Fig. 6.13) exhibited its characteristic oxidation and reduction current magnitude, which is typical behavior of bare CCY. The magnitude of oxidation response current for MWCNTs/CCY nanocomposite increases to ~412 μA. The results evident that incorporation of MWCNTs onto CCY with high concentration was enhanced the electro catalytic behavior of MWCNTs.

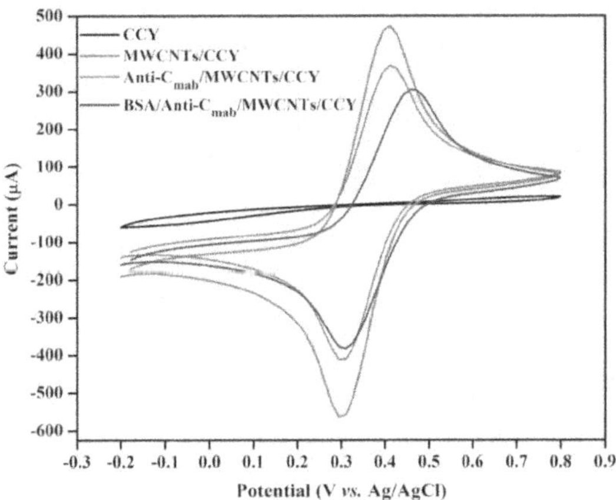

Fig. 6.13 CV analysis of step wise fabrication of BSA/Anti-C$_{mab}$/MWCNTs/CCY immunoelectrode in PBS (10 mM, pH 7.0)

The response current peaks were found to be stable and reversible at particular scan rate. The magnitude of the electrochemical current response was reduced to ~368 μA after the immobilization of Anti-C$_{mab}$ onto MWCNTs/CCY nanocomposite electrode. The decreased current response was due to hindrance in electron transport caused by the insulating nature of antibodies. Furthermore, the magnitude of current response of BSA/AntiC$_{mab}$/MWCNTs/CCY immunoelectrode was observed to be lower than that of Anti-C$_{mab}$/MWCNTs/CCY electrode. Decrease in response current is attributed to the hindrance in charge transformation due to the insulating behavior of BSA via blocking of non-specific binding cites.

6.4.3 Effect of pH

In the Fig. 6.14a, it was observed that the magnitude of the electrochemical current response of BSA/Anti-C$_{mab}$/MWCNTs/CCY immunoelectrode decreased while increasing pH from 5.0 to 6.0. Further increasing the pH upto 7.0, the redox peak current increased. However, beyond the pH 7.0 the current responses gradually decreased as shown in Fig. 6.14b. It might because the immunoelectrode lost its electrochemical activity in the base supporting electrolyte medium. So, the immunosensor response towards cortisol was found better at pH 7.0. Thus, pH 7.0 was chosen as the optimized working electrolyte pH.

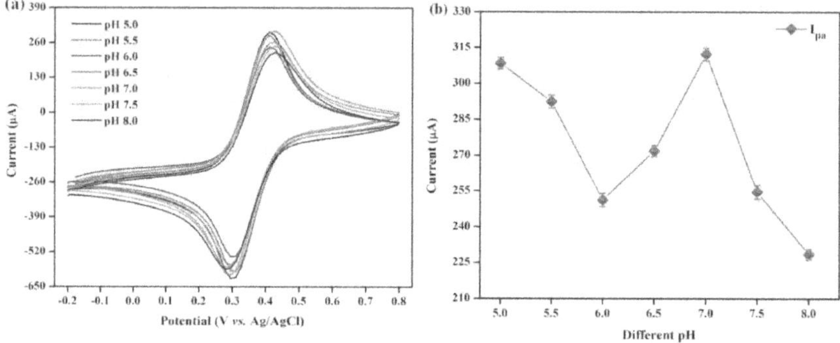

Fig. 6.14 (a) CV analysis of the BSA/Anti-C$_{mab}$/MWCNTs/CCY immunoelectrode as a function of pH from 5.0 to 8.0 and (b) Linear plots of peak current *vs.* pH values

6.4.4. Effect of scan rate

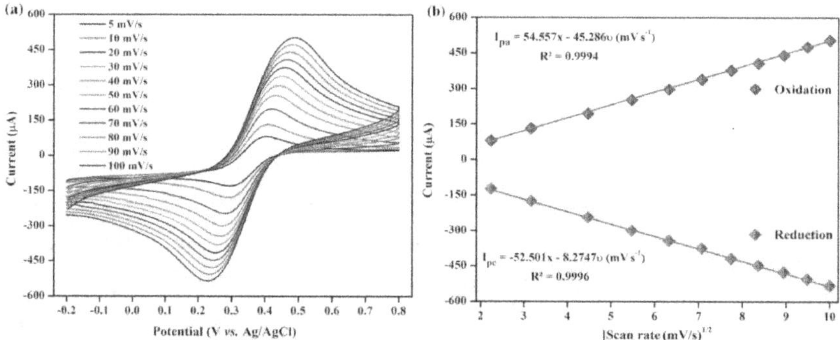

Fig. 6.15 (a) CV analysis of the BSA/Anti-C$_{mab}$/MWCNTs/CCY immunoelectrode as a function of scan rates (5 to 100 mV/s) in PBS (10 mM, pH 7.0) and (b) Linear plot of the oxidation and reduction peak currents *vs.* square root of scan rates

The effect of scan rate (5-100 mV/s) on the electrochemical behavior of BSA/Anti-C_{mab}/MWCNTs/CCY immunoelectrode was studied and presented in Fig. 6.15a. The magnitude of electrochemical current response of immunoelectrode was linearly dependent on the scan rate exhibiting an almost linear relationship (shown in Fig. 6.15b) and the corresponding equation (Eq. 6.1 and 6.2) are follow,

$$I_{pa}(\mu A) = 54.557x - 45.286\upsilon \ (mV/s); \ R^2 = 0.9994 \qquad -------(Eq.\,6.1)$$

$$I_{pc}(\mu A) = -52.501x - 8.2747\upsilon \ (mV/s); \ R^2 = 0.9996 \qquad -------(Eq.\,6.2)$$

The observed well-defined stable redox peaks as a function of scan rate suggested that it was a surface-controlled electrochemical process. The separation of peaks suggested that the process was not perfectly reversible; however, stable redox peak current and position during repeated scans at a particular scan rate exhibited a quasi-reversible process.

6.4.5 Cortisol response studies of BSA/Anti-C_{mab}/MWCNTs/CCY immunoelectrode by CV

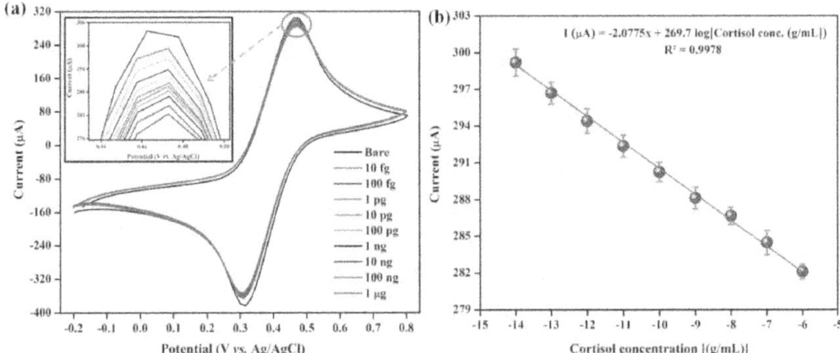

Fig. 6.16 (a) Electrochemical studies of BSA/Anti-C_{mab}/MWCNTs/CCY immunoelectrode as a function of cortisol concentration varied from 10 fg to 1 μg in PBS (10 mM, pH 7.0) and (b) Linear plot between electrochemical peak current response and logarithm of cortisol concentration

The electrochemical response current studies of BSA/Anti-C_{mab}/MWCNTs/CCY immunoelectrode has been studied using CV technique in triplet set using PBS

(10 mM, pH 7.0) at scan rate of 50 mV/s by varying the cortisol concentration ranging from 10 fg to 1 µg. Fig. 6.16a, depicts that the electrochemical current response decreased as a function of increasing cortisol concentration. Decrease in response current was attributed to the formation of insulating immunocomplex between Anti-C_{mab} and cortisol which hindered electron transport.

A calibration curve between the oxidation current response and logarithm of cortisol concentration has been plotted and shown in Fig. 6.16b, which revealed a linear correlation up to 1 µg and given in the equation (Eq. 6.3),

$$\Delta I\ (\mu A) = -2.0775x + 269.70\ [Cortisol\ conc.\ (g/mL);\ R^2 = 0.9978\ ---(Eq.6.3)$$

The immunosensor exhibited a linear detection range from 10 fg to 1 µg with a regression coefficient (R^2) value of 0.997. The detection limit of the fabricated BSA/Anti-C_{mab}/MWCNTs/CCY immunosensor was calculated as 2.69 fg/mL by using standard equation (Eq. 2.8).

6.4.6 Cortisol response studies of BSA/Anti-C_{mab}/MWCNTs/CCY immunoelectrode by DPV

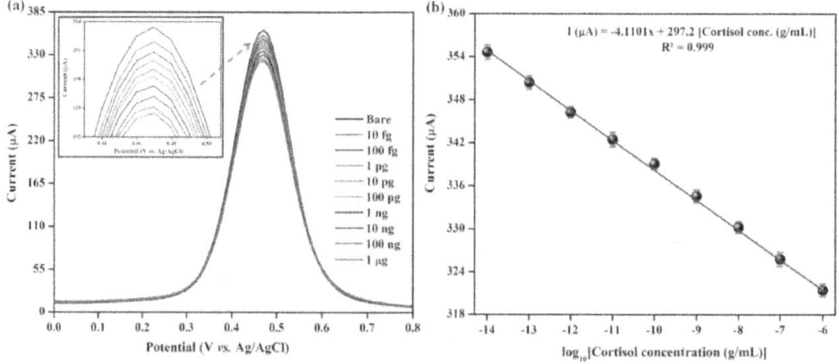

Fig. 6.17 (a) DPV analysis of the BSA/Anti-C_{mab}/MWCNTs/CCY immunoelectrode as a function of cortisol concentration varied from 10 fg to 1 µg in PBS (10 mM, pH 7.0) and (b) Linear plot between electrochemical peak current response and logarithm of cortisol concentration

The insulating behavior of cortisol binding was investigated for various cortisol concentrations (Fig. 6.17a) using DPV method. It is clear that increasing cortisol concentration the electrochemical current decreased linearly in the range 10 fg – 1 µg, followed the linear equation (Eq. 6.4),

$$\Delta I \ (\mu A) = -4.1101x + 297.2 \ [Cortisol \ conc. \ (g/mL); \ R^2 = 0.999 \ - - - -(Eq. 6.4)$$

In Fig. 6.17b, illustrated the linear calibration curve obtained between the logarithm of cortisol concentration and the magnitude of electrochemical response current exposed the good linear range from 10 fg to 1 µg with a correlation coefficient of 0.999 with detection limit of 0.56 fg/mL.

6.4.7 Interference studies

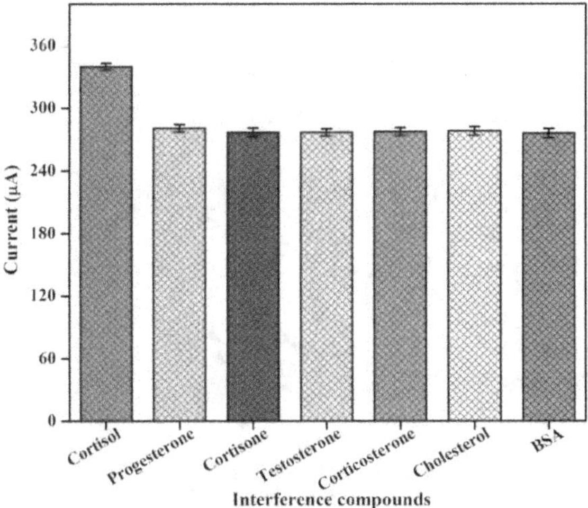

Fig. 6.18 Interference studies of BSA/Anti-C$_{mab}$/MWCNTs/CCY immunoelectrode towards Progesterone, Testosterone, Cortisone, Corticosterone, Cholesterol and BSA with respect to cortisol (100 ng/mL) in PBS (10 mM, pH 7.0)

Interference studies were conducted by testing the BSA/Anti-C$_{mab}$/MWCNTs/CCY immunoelectrode with interferents through CV analysis. The interferents used in the present study were progesterone, testosterone, corticosterone, cortisone, cholesterol and BSA of each 100 ng/mL towards cortisol. In Fig. 6.18, the observed peak current responses of BSA/Anti-C$_{mab}$/MWCNTs/CCY electrode towards cortisol (100 ng/mL) in presence of interferents haven't showed higher difference. It further assured that the current responses after the simultaneous addition of interferents species, the prepared electrode retained its electrochemical response almost 80 % of its actual value in the absence of interferences.

6.4.8 Stability, repeatability and reproducibility studies

The stability of the MWCNTs/CCY immunoelectrode was studied periodically towards the detection of 100 ng/mL of cortisol for four weeks. The BSA/Anti-C$_{mab}$/MWCNTs/CCY immunoelectrode retained 95.20% of the initial current response of cortisol after the storage at 4 °C, which indicated that the prepared binder free immunoelectrode has a better stability. Also, the stability of MWCNTs/CCY based was investigated by measuring the current response using CV method for 1000 cycles in 10 mM PBS as shown in Fig. 6.19. The RSD values were calculated from the current responses obtained for MWCNTs/CCY of 3.42% which indicating the good stability of the developed electrode.

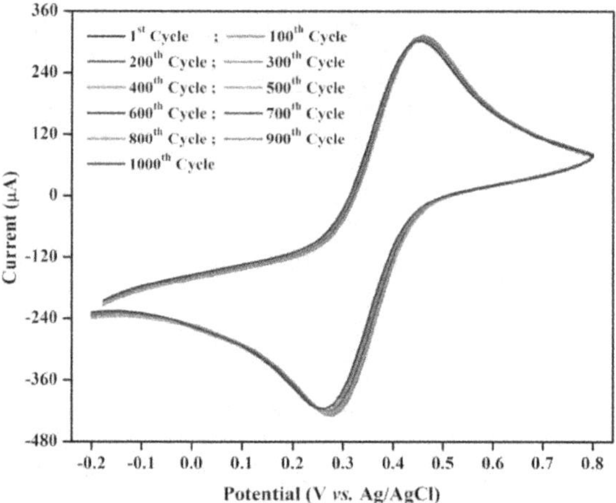

Fig. 6.19 The stability analysis of MWCNTs/CCY immunoelectrode for 1000 cycles in 10 mM PBS

The RSD value of 3.8 % was found for 10 measurements of 100 ng/mL of cortisol by single BSA/Anti-C$_{mab}$/MWCNTs/CCY immunoelectrode which ensured its repeatability. The five BSA/Anti-C$_{mab}$/MWCNTs/CCY immunoelectrodes were prepared independently and subjected to the cortisol detection to calculate the reproducibility of the modified electrode. The RSD of measurements was 3.6 % for cortisol, which was exposed the better reproducibility of binder free BSA/Anti-C$_{mab}$/MWCNTs/CCY immunoelectrode. Thus, these results indicated the prepared immunosensor has good reproducibility and electrochemically stable to be employed in the biosensor applications.

6.4.9 Real sample analysis

We further examined the practicability of prepared immunosensor through analyzing real sweat samples and the results are given in Table 6.1. Herein, CV method was used to detect the cortisol level in human sweat. The RSD of the proposed immunosensor from 3.25 % to 5.13 % and the recovery rates of the samples ranged between 95.46 % and 104.73 %. The significant recoveries attained in various sweat samples for the determination of cortisol.

Table 6.1 Comparison of sweat cortisol estimated using chemiluminescence immunoassay and MWCNTs/CCY based electrochemical immunosensor

Samples	CLIA method (ng/mL)	MWCNTs/CCY immunosensor				
		Measured (ng/mL)*	Added (ng/mL)	Found (ng/mL)*	RSD (%)	Recovery (%)
1	20	22.34	50	73.75	3.245	101.94
2	28	33.67	50	81.54	3.654	104.73
3	32	34.98	50	81.13	5.126	95.46
4.	57	62.75	50	110.64	4.323	98.12
5.	61	58.12	50	110.11	3.556	101.84

*** The average value of three successive experiments.**

Also, the obtained results were validated using commercially available CILA method (Fig. 6.20). The results obtained from both the techniques are summarized in Table 6.1.

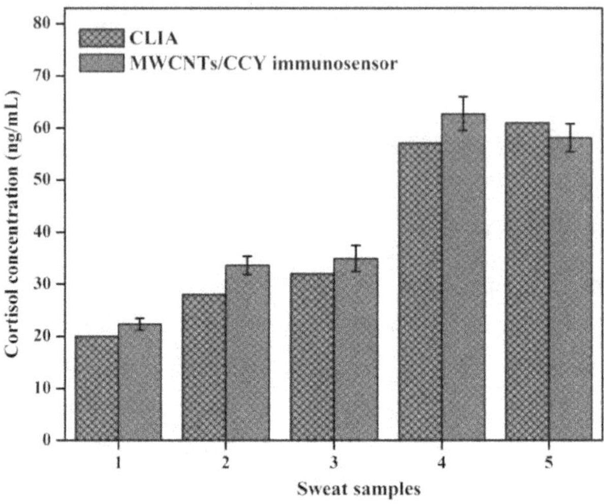

Fig. 6.20 Comparison graph of sweat cortisol estimated using chemiluminescence immunoassay and MWCNTs/CCY based electrochemical immunosensor

6.5 Conclusions

In summary, we have constructed binder free MWCNTs/CCY based immunoelectrode for sensitive detection of cortisol in human sweat. For this, the functionalized MWCNTs were integrated on CCY by simple dip coating method. The structural, morphological, electrical, mechanical and electrochemical activity results exhibited improved immunosensing properties of MWCNTs. CV studies exposed a stable current response towards cortisol of prepared electrode during repeated scanning in PBS solution of pH 7.0. The CV and DPV results showed that the cortisol detection was found up to 1 µg, with a detection limit of ~2.7 and 0.5 fg/mL in addition with notable anti-interference ability. Nevertheless, of its improved conductivity and mechanical stability, the surface wettability study showed the hydrophobic nature of MWCNTs integrated fiber compared to analyzed metal oxides. This might inferior in the sweat based cortisol detection. Thus, we aimed to incorporate Fe_2O_3 on its surface and analyzed the immunosensor performance of the resultant hybrid. The results are discussed in following chapter.

References

1. J. H. Lehman, M. Terrones, E. Mansfield, K. E. Hurst, V. Meunier, Evaluating the characteristics of multiwall carbon nanotubes, *Carbon,* **49** (2011) 2581–2602.

2. A. Aqel, K. M.M. Abou El-Nour, R. A.A. Ammar, A. A. Warthan, Carbon nanotubes, science and technology part (I) structure, synthesis and characterization, *Arab. J. Chem.,* **5** (2012) 1–23.

3. Y. Yang, M. C. Gupta, K.L Dudley, R. W. Lawrence, Novel carbon nanotube-Polystyrene foam composites for electromagnetic interference shielding, *Nano Lett.,* **5** (2005) 2131–2134.

4. X. Shui, and D. D. L. Chung, Magnetic properties of nickel filament polymer-matrix composites, *J. Electron. Mater.,* **25** (1996) 930–934.

5. L. L. Wang, B. K. Tay, K. Y. See, Z. Sun, L. K. Tan, D. Lua, Electromagnetic interference shielding effectiveness of carbon-based materials prepared by screen printing, *Carbon,* **47** (2009) 1905–1910.

6. Z. Chen, C. Xu, C. Ma, W. Ren, H. M. Cheng, Lightweight and flexible graphene foam composites for high-performance electromagnetic interference shielding, *Adv. Mater.,* **25** (2013) 1296–1300.

7. T. W. Lee, S. E. Lee, Y. G. Jeong, Carbon nanotube/cellulose papers with high performance in electric heating and electromagnetic interference shielding, *Compos. Sci. Technol.,* **131** (2016) 77–87.

8. F. L. Michael De Volder, S. H. Tawfick, R. H. Baughman, A. J. Hart, Carbon nanotubes: Present and future commercial applications, *Science,* **339** (2013) 535-539.

9. Y. Ueki, T.Aoki, K. Ueda, M. Shibahara, Thermophysical properties of carbon-based material nanofluid, *Mater. Sci.,* **113** (2017) 1130-1134.

10. S. Iijima, Helical microtubules of graphitic carbon, *Nature,* **354** (1991) 56–58.

11. G. Yarlagadda, G. Solasa, R. Boanapalli, P. Paladugu, S. G. Babu, Three-dimensional finite element (FE) model for armchair and zigzag type single-walled carbon nanotube, *Int J Sci Res.,* **3** (2013) 1-9.

12. C. Klumpp, K. Kostarelos, M. Prato, A. Bianco, Functionalized carbon nanotubes as emerging nanovectors for the delivery of therapeutics, *Biochem Biophys Acta*, **1758** (2006) 404-412.

13. D. Danailov, P. Keblinski, S. Nayak, P. M. Ajayan, Bending properties of carbon nanotubes encapsulating solid nanowires, *J Nano Sci Nanotechnol.*, **2** (2002) 503-507.

14. B. Zhang, Q. Chen, H. Tang, Q. Xie, M. Ma, L. Tan, Y. Zhang, S. Yao, Characterization and biomolecule immobilization on the biocompatible multi-walled carbon nanotubes generated by functionalization with polyamidoamine dendrimers, *Colloids Surf B Biointerfaces*, **80** (2010) 18-25.

15. V. Rastogi, P. Yadav, S. Bhattacharya, A. K. Mishra, N. Verma, A. Verma, J. K. Pandit, Carbon Nanotubes: An Emerging Drug Carrier for Targeting Cancer Cells, *Drug Delivery*, **670815** (2014) 1-23.

16. Z. H. Xia, P. R. Guduru, W. A. Curtin, Enhancing mechanical properties of multiwall carbon nanotubes via sp3 interwall bridging, *Phys. Rev. Lett.*, **98** (2007) 245501- 245504.

17. S. Y. Madan, N. Naderi, O. Dissanayake, A. Tan, A. M Seifalian, A new era of cancer treatment: carbon nanotubes as drug delivery tools, *Int J Nanomedicine*, **6** (2011) 2963- 2979.

18. E. G. U. Cayetan, F. Avilés, J. V. C. Rodríguez, R. Schönfelder, A. Bachmatiuk, M. H. Rümmeli, F. Rubio, M. P. G. Amador, G. J. Cruz, Influence of nanotube physicochemical properties on the decoration of multiwall carbon nanotubes with magnetic particles, *J Nanopart Res.*, **16** (2014) 2192 (1-13).

19. P. Pandey and M. Dahiya, Carbon nanotubes: Types, methods of preparation and applications, *Int J Pharm Sci Res.*, **1** (2016) 15-21.

20. C. Journet and P. Bernier, Production of carbon nanotubes, *Appl. Phys.*, **67** (1998) 1–9.

21. N. Saifuddin, A. Z. Raziah, and A. R. Junizah, Carbon Nanotubes: A review on structure and their interaction with proteins, *J. Chem.*, **676815** (2013) 1- 18.

22. K. Sarangdevot and B. S. Sonigara, The Wondrous World of Carbon Nanotubes, a review of current carbon nanotube technologies, *J Chem Pharm Res.*, **7** (2015) 916-933

23. M. A. Jie, J. A. Wang, C. J. Tsai, R. Nussino, M. A. Buyong, Diameters of single walled carbon nanotubes (SWCNTs) and related nanochemistry and nanobiology, *Front Mater Sci China,* **4** (2010) 17-28.

24. C. H. See and A. T. Harris, A review of carbon nanotube synthesis via fluidized-bed chemical vapor deposition, *Ind. Eng. Chem. Res.,* **46** (2007) 997–1012.

25. K. Varshney, Carbon nanotubes: A review on synthesis, properties and applications, *Int J Eng Res Gen Sci.,* **2** (2014) 660-677.

26. B. S. Shim, W. Chen, C. Doty, C. Xu, N. A. Kotov, Smart electronic yarns and wearable fabrics for human biomonitoring made by carbon nanotube coating with polyelectrolytes, *Nano Lett.,* **8** (2008) 4151-4157.

27. S.P. Sharma, S.C. Lakkad, Effect of CNTs growth on carbon fibers on the tensile strength of CNTs grown carbon fiber-reinforced polymer matrix composites, *Composites: Part A,* **42** (2011) 8–15.

28. E. T. Thostenson, W. Z. Li, D. Z. Wang, Z. F. Ren, T. W. Chou, Carbon nanotube/ carbon fiber hybrid multiscale composites, *J. Appl. Phys.,* **91** (2002) 6034-6037.

29. X. Wu, H. Xie, Q. Deng, H. X. Wang, H. Sheng, Y.X. Yin, W. X. Zhou, R.L. Li, Yu-G. Guo, Three-dimensional carbon nanotubes forest/carbon cloth as an efficient electrode for Li-polysulfide batteries, *ACS Appl. Mater. Interfaces,* **18** (2017) 1553-1561.

30. S. Wang and R. A. W. Dryfe, Graphene oxide-assisted deposition of carbon nanotubes on carbon cloth as advanced binder-free electrodes for flexible supercapacitors, *J. Mater. Chem. A,* **1** (2013) 5279–5283.

31. M. M. Barsana, R. C. Carvalhoa, Y. Zhong, X. Sunb, C. M. A. Bretta, Carbon nanotube modified carbon cloth electrodes: Characterisation and application as biosensors, *Electrochim. Acta,* **85** (2012) 203– 209.

32. L. Wang and K. J Loh, Wearable carbon nanotube-based fabric sensors for monitoring human physiological performance, *Smart Mater. Struct.,* **26** (2017) 055018 (1-11).

33. C. Tlili, N. V. Myunga, V. Shettyb, A. Mulchandania, Label-free, chemiresistor immunosensor for stress biomarker cortisol in saliva, *Biosens. Bioelectron,* **26** (2011) 4382– 4386.

34. M. M. Guzmán, L. Agüí, A. G. Cortés and P. Y. Sedeño, J. M. Pingarrón, Gold nanoparticles/carbon nanotubes/ionic liquid microsized paste electrode for the determination of cortisol and androsterone hormones, *J Solid State Electrochem*, **17** (2013) 1591–1599.

35. P. Manickam, R. E. Fernandez, Y. Umasankar, M. Gurusamy, F. Arizaleta, G. Urizar, S. Bhansali, Salivary cortisol analysis using metalloporphyrins and multi-walled carbon nanotubes nanocomposite functionalized electrodes, *Sens. Actuator B-Chem*, **274** (2018) 47-53.

36. H. Qi, J. Liu, Y. Deng, S. Gao, E. Mäder, Cellulose fibres with carbon nanotube networks for water sensing, *J. Mater. Chem. A*, **2** (2014) 5541-5547.

37. D. Gopi, E. Shinyjoy, M. Sekar, M. Surendiran, L. Kavitha, T.S.S. Kumar, *Corros. Sci.*, **73** (2013) 321-330.

38. J. Feng, H. Xia, F. Mao, Alignment of Ag nanowires on glass sheet by dip coating technique, *J Alloys Compd.*, **735** (2018) 607-612 .

39. M. E. Spotnitz, D. Ryan and H. A. Stone, Dip coating for the alignment of carbon nanotubes on curved surfaces, *J. Mater. Chem.*, **14** (2004) 1299 – 1302.

40. J. Miao, F.X. Xiao, H.B. Yang, S.Y. Khoo, J. Chen, Z. Fan, Y. Hsu, H.M. Chen, H. Zhang, B. Liu, Hierarchical Ni-Mo-S nanosheets on carbon fiber cloth: A flexible electrode for efficient hydrogen generation in neutral electrolyte, *Sci. Adv.*, **1** (2015) 1–14.

41. N. R. Chodankar, S. H. Ji, D. H. Kim, Surface modified carbon cloth via nitrogen plasma for supercapacitor applications, *J. Electrochem. Soc.*, **165** (2018) 2446-2450.

42. S. Madhu, P. Manickam, M. Pierre, S. Bhansali, P. Nagamony, V. Chinnuswamy, Nanostructured SnO2 integrated conductive fabrics as binder-free electrode for neurotransmitter detection, *Sens. Actuators, A* **269** (2018) 401–411.

43. V. Eswaraiah, V. Sankaranarayanan, S. Ramaprabhu, Inorganic nanotubes reinforced polyvinylidene fluoride composites as low-cost electromagnetic interference shielding materials, *Nanoscale Res. Lett.*, **37** (2011) 1-12.

44. Z. S. Cao, Li Qiu, Y. Yang, Y. K. Chen, X. Liu, The surface modifications of multi-walled carbon nanotubes for multi-walled carbon nanotube/poly (ether ether ketone) composites, *Appl. Surf. Sci.,* **353** (2015) 873-881.

45. S. De, S. Niranjana, B.S. Satyanarayanan, K. Mohan Rao, Raman spectroscopy and conductivity variation of nanocluster carbon fiber films grown using a room temperature based cathodic arc process, *Sci. Iran.,* **18** (2011) 797-803.

46. Y. Wang, S. Serrano, J. J. Santiago, Aviler-Raman characterization of carbon nanofibers prepared using electrospinning, *Synth Met.,* **138** (2003) 423-427.

47. S. Luo, Y. Wang, G. Wang, K. Wang, Z. Wang, C. Zhang, B. Wang, Y. Luo, L. Li, T. Liu, CNT Enabled Co-braided smart fabrics: A new route for noninvasive, highly sensitive & large area monitoring of composites, *Sci. Rep.,* **7** (2017) 44056 (1-10).

48. R. C. Zhuang, T. L. Doan, J. W. Liu, J. Zhang, S. L. Gao, E. Mader, Multi-functional multi-walled carbon nanotube-jute fibres and composites, *Carbon,* **49** (2011) 2683 –2692.

49. S. J. P. Gamage, K. Yang, R. Braveenth, K. Raagulan, H. S. Kim, Y. S. Lee, C. M. Yang, J. J. Moon, K. Y. Chai, MWCNT coated Free-standing Carbon Fiber Fabric for Enhanced Performance in EMI Shielding with a higher absolute EMI SE, *Materials,* **10** (2017) 1350 (1-12).

50. C. F. Wang, W. Y. Chen, H. Z. Cheng, S. L. Fu, Pressure proof superhydrophobic films from flexible carbon nanotube/polymer coatings, *J. Phys. Chem. C,* **114** (2010) 15607–11.

51. N. B. Duong, S. L. You, L. Z. Huang, H. Yang, Carbon nanotubes modified carbon cloth cathode electrode for self-pumping enzymatic biofuel cell, *J. Renew. Sustain. Energy,* **8748731** (2018) 1-8.

52. F. D. Nicola, P. Castrucci1, M. Scarselli, F. Nanni, I. Cacciotti, M. D. Crescenzi, Super-hydrophobic multi-walled carbon nanotube coatings for stainless steel, *Nanotechnology,* **26** (2015) 145701 (1-6).

Chapter VII

Fe₂O₃ Nanoparticles Decorated MWCNTS Coated Carbon Yarn for the Synergetic Detection of Stress Biomarker

Highlights

φ α-Fe$_2$O$_3$ wrapped on the outer surface of MWCNTs/CCY to form immunosensor.

φ A binder free Fe$_2$O$_3$/MWCNTs/CCY was exhibited superior electrochemical properties towards analyte cortisol.

φ The target molecule was quantified with broad detection range and low detection limit.

φ The composite provided combinational benefits to be used as a sensitive, selective platform towards cortisol in human sweat samples.

φ The validation of the sensor performance of developed immunoelectrode with CILA method assured its pertinent in real time.

Graphical illustration of immobilization and electrochemical immunosensing of cortisol on hydrothermally derived Fe₂O₃ /MWCNTs/CCY with possible redox mechanism

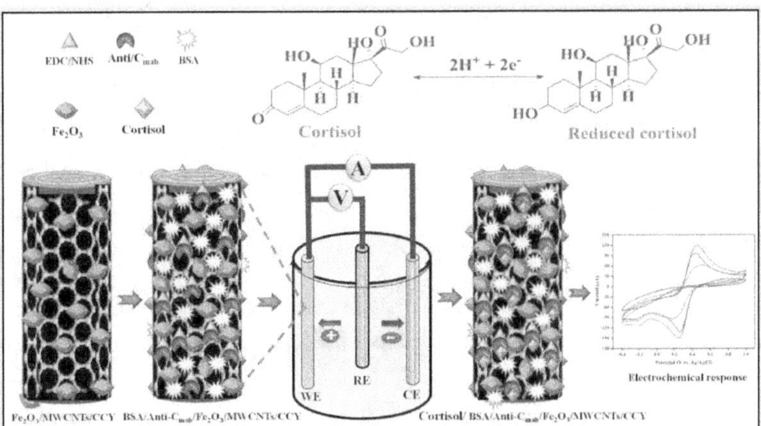

7.1 Introduction

Nanocomposites are solid materials that have several phase domains and at least one of these domains has a nanoscale structure. The materials can have novel chemical and physical properties that depend on the morphology and interfacial characteristics of the constituents materials [1].

As a promising class of materials, CNTs based nanocomposites have attracted considerable research attention in recent years owing to their potential applications in catalysis, sensors, hydrogen storage and power storage devices, etc. Carbon-based nanomaterials, including single-and multi-walled CNTs, fullerenes, and graphene, are currently being the attractive nanomaterials from application perspectives. Since their discovery in 1991 by Sumio Iijima, carbon nanotubes have been intensively studied. These carbon materials widely used as supporting matrices to develop several functional nanomaterials and hybrids. These novel materials are generally prepared by adding a secondary phase (i.e., functional components) to the external surfaces of either SWCNTs or MWCNTs [2, 3]. Structurally, these materials have a phase (or compositional) difference across the radial direction and a constant concentric arrangement of each participating component along the axial direction [4, 5].

There has been numerous way of preparing these kinds of nanocomposites which include the conventional impregnation method, hydrothermal method, dip coating, sol-gel technique, electrochemical reduction, chemical vapor deposition and micro-emulsion techniques. These techniques are used to introduce active inorganic components such as metals, transition metals and their oxides and sulfides such as Au, Ag, Pt, Rh, Pd, TiO_2, SnO_2, Fe_2O_3, ZnO, ZnS, and NiS onto the CNTs [6-11]. To improve interfacial adhesion between an additional component and CNTs, surface treatments such as acid-assisted oxidation and ultrasonication have been applied from which new surface functional groups, or additional covalent and/or non-covalent interconnectivity to the secondary phases, may be provoked [12].

Recently, Nan Yan *et al.,* reported that the Fe_2O_3 nanoparticles wrapped on the MWCNTs novel hybrid nanostructures for the enhanced lithium storage capability [6]. This hybrid nanostructure exhibited a discharge capacity of 515 mAh g^{-1}, after 50 cycles as anode electrode for LIBs, while the capacity is calculated as 1147 mAhg^{-1} based on the mass ratio of Fe$_2$O$_3$ nanoparticles. Such a superior property could be attributed to the unique structure of MWCNTs wrapping which not only accommodates the large volume difference but also enhanced the overall conductivity.

Xu Chen *et al.,* (2019) α-Fe$_2$O$_3$ nanoparticles/MWCNTs hybrids were successfully prepared via a facile one-step hydrothermal method. The conductivity of the MWCNTs enhanced and provided space for stress and strain during volume expansion of α-Fe$_2$O$_3$ semiconductor as the anode for LIBs. The composite showed remarkable electrochemical performance when it was used as the electrodes of coin cells. The α-Fe$_2$O$_3$ electrode with 50 wt% of MWCNTs retained its capacity of 816.8 mAh g^{-1} after 50 cycles at the current density of 200 mA g^{-1}. Furthermore, the flexible carbon nanofiber paper (CNP) has also been investigated as a novel current collector in LIBs and the capacity of free-standing α-Fe$_2$O$_3$/50 wt% MWCNTs/CNP hybrids electrode can retained 467.2 mAh g^{-1} after 50 cycles under the current density of changes from 2500 mA g^{-1} to 200 mA g^{-1}. Finally they concluded, the MWCNTs improved cycle performance, enhanced reversible capacities and rate capability of MWCNTs/α-Fe$_2$O$_3$ anodes could attributed the inherent conducting network, shorten electron pathway and faster reaction kinetics [13].

Also, X. R. Lin *et al.,* (2018) described the preparation of MWCNTs/Fe$_2$O$_3$ nanocomposites and its application in the electrochemical detection of nitrite. The CV results showed that the Fe$_2$O$_3$/MWCNTs modified GCE presented excellent electrochemical activity in the presence of 1 mM nitrite in a 0.1 M PBS compared to the Fe$_2$O$_3$ and MWCNTs-modified GCE. Electrochemical studies showed that the composite exhibited a low detection limit (0.1 μM) and a wide linear range (10–1000 μM) to nitrite with a fast current response. In addition, the modified electrode showed long-term stability and excellent reproducibility. The prepared electrochemical sensor demonstrated significant selectivity, sensitivity and it was also showed good performance in real sample analysis [14].

Regarding the cortisol detection, only B. Sun *et al.,* (2017) developed sensitive competitive electrochemical immunosensor for the detection of cortisol was successfully developed based on gold nanoparticles and magnetic (Fe$_3$O$_4$) functionalized reduced graphene oxide (AuNPs/MrGO). A variety of cortisol loaded in the AuNPs/MrGO with large specific surface area and good bioactivity to assemble the basic electrode (Cor/AuNPs/MrGO/Nafion@GCE), which was characterized by the CV and EIS studies proved its excellent electrical conductivity. The immunosensor exhibited admirable analytical performance for the detection of cortisol range from 0.1 to 1000 ng/mL with a detection limit of 0.05 ng/mL. Also, compared the developed immunosensor with commercially available ELISA and concluded the present strategy provides a novel and convenient method for clinical determination of cortisol [15].

In this *chapter VII*, the preparation of nanocomposite based immunosensing platform for the binder free electrochemical detection of cortisol was described. Further, the electrochemical analysis was based on antigen–antibody interaction that provides the specific and selective detection of a stress biomarker. The α-Fe$_2$O$_3$ nanostructures *(Optimized in Chapter IV)* are used to decorate on MWCNTs/CCY *(Optimized in Chapter VI)* through hydrothermal method to develop hybrid nanocomposites. For the first time, hydrothermally deposited α-Fe$_2$O$_3$@MWCNTs hybrid nanocomposite is exploited for the immobilization of monoclonal Anti-C$_{mab}$ to realize a binder free electrochemical immunosensing performance for cortisol detection.

7.2 Materials and methods

7.2.1 Chemicals and reagents

All other reagents were of analytical grade and were used as received without further purification.

7.2.2 Decoration of α-Fe$_2$O$_3$ on MWCNTs coated CCY

In typical preparation of Fe$_2$O$_3$ on MWCNTs/CCY nanocomposites, 0.22 g of FeCl$_3$.6H$_2$O and 1 g of the Pluronic f127 were dissolved in 30 mL of DI water to form a homogeneous solution under 30 min continuously stirring and then transferred to a 70 mL Teflon-lined autoclave. The MWCNTs/CCY *(Optimized in chapter VI)* was immersed into the prepared solution and heated at 180 °C for 12 hours. After hydrothermal process, the obtained yarns was washed with DD water and ethanol for several times and then dried at 60 °C overnight.

7.2.3 Immobilization of Anti-C_{mab} onto Fe$_2$O$_3$/MWCNTs/CCY

Standard process, reported in previous chapters, has been utilized to immobilize Anti-C_{mab} onto Fe$_2$O$_3$/MWCNTs/CCY electrode. Anti-C_{mab} was covalently bound on nanocomposites via EDC/NHS chemistry between amine group of MWCNTs/Fe$_2$O$_3$ and COOH group of Anti-C_{mab}. The volume of Anti-C_{mab} for immobilization was optimized and best results were observed when 80 μL of 2 μg/mL was used for surface modification. A consistent response current was obtained after the incubation period of 120 mins followed by PBS washing. Non-binding sites on Anti-C_{mab}/Fe$_2$O$_3$/MWCNTs/CCY immunoelectrode were blocked by 30 min of incubation in a 60 μg/mL BSA solution in PBS (10 mM, pH 7.0). The fabricated BSA/Anti-C_{mab}/Fe$_2$O$_3$/MWCNTs/CCY immunoelectrodes were washed several times with PBS solution and stored at 4 °C when not in use.

7.3 Results and discussion

7.3.1 XRD analysis of CCY, MWCNTs/CCY and Fe$_2$O$_3$/MWCNTs/CCY

The crystallographic structures of the hybrid nanocomposite material were analyzed by XRD and the results are shown in Fig. 7.1. The results showed the diffraction peaks of CCY and MWCNT/CCY at ~$2\theta = 26°$ and 43.2° corresponding to the (002) and (100) respectively [16, 17]. Compared to the CCY, the MWCNTs integrated CCY confirmed the sharp peak with increased intensity which endorsed the uniform coating without any impurities [18, 19]. Furthermore, Fe$_2$O$_3$/MWCNTs/CCY composite showed the diffraction peaks of Fe$_2$O$_3$ at 24.29°, 33.38° (major), 35.83°, 41.11°, 49.78°, 54.45°, 58.05°, 62.87° and 64.39° can be obviously found, which indexed to the (012), (104), (113), (024), (116), (018), (214) and (330) planes of hematite (α-Fe$_2$O$_3$) nanoparticles and the outcomes were in accordance with standard JCPDS card no. 84-0309 [Rhomb-centered rhombohedral system, space group: R3c (167)] along with carbon peaks [10, 21, 22]. No peaks for impurities were detected, indicating that the hydrothermal method used in this study is responsible for the formation of the Fe$_2$O$_3$ on MWCNTs/CCY composite with high purity [14].

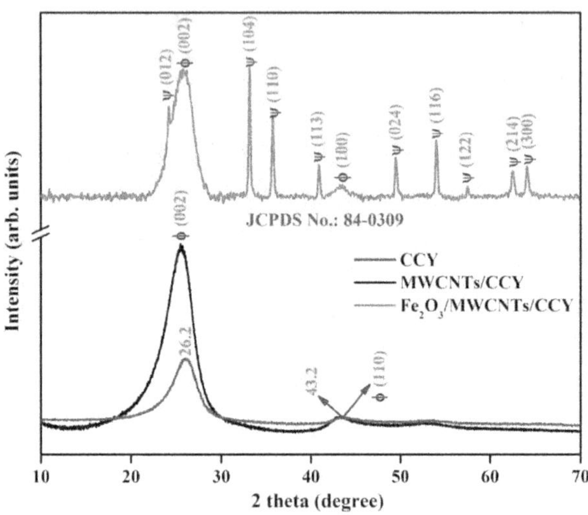

Fig. 7.1 X-ray diffraction patterns of CCY, MWCNTs/CCY and Fe₂O₃/MWCNTs/CCY

7.3.2 FT-IR spectra of CCY, MWCNTs/CCY and Fe₂O₃/MWCNTs/CCY

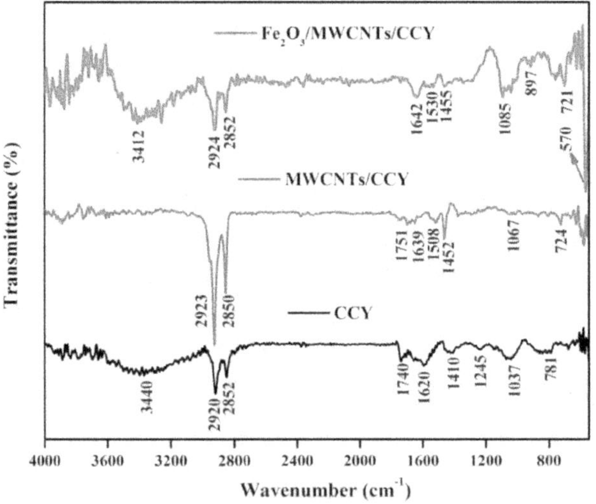

Fig. 7.2 FT-IR spectra of CCY, MWCNTs/CCY and Fe₂O₃/MWCNTs/CCY

For the understanding of the successful coating of Fe_2O_3/MWCNTs/CCY composite, the chemical bonds present in CCY, MWCNTs/CCY and Fe_2O_3/MWCNTs/CCY were studied using FT-IR in the wavelength range of 500 to 4000 cm^{-1}. The Fig. 7.2 shows the IR spectra of uncoated carbon fiber in which it is possible to identify absorption bands such as 3440 cm^{-1}, that could be assigned to the axial deformation of O-H; 781, 2920 and 2882 cm^{-1} were attributed to the axial deformation of C-H present in the structure. The band at 1620 cm^{-1}, that was arouse from the stretching vibration of C=C. In addition 1245 cm^{-1}, related to the stretching vibration C-O-C and at 1037 cm^{-1}, that could be referred to the aliphatic-aromatic linkage [23, 24]. After the dip coating of MWCNTs on CCY, the intensity of the peaks of C-H groups (724, 2850 and 2923 cm^{-1}), C=C (1452 cm^{-1}), C-O (1067 cm^{-1}) were substantially increased, indicating that the huge amount MWCNTs successfully coated on CCY [25].

Moreover in the Fig. 7.2, approximately the same peaks were observed in spectrum of MWCNTs/Fe_2O_3/CCY hybrid in the wave numbers 721, 1085, 1455, 1642, 2852, 2924 and 3412 cm^{-1}, respectively. In addition to this, the peak in 570 cm^{-1}, 897 cm^{-1} is attributed due to the stretching and bending vibration modes of Fe–O and Fe-O-H; the enhanced intensity for Fe–O is indicative of the iron loading in MWCNTs/CCY [26, 27]. From the FT-IR results, we confirmed that the Fe_2O_3 were decorated onto the MWCNTs/CCY surface uniformly.

7.3.3 Raman spectra of CCY, MWCNTs/CCY and Fe₂O₃/MWCNTs/CCY

Raman spectroscopy was used to study the graphitization degree and crystalline quality of the Fe_2O_3 decorated over MWCNTs/CCY. As shown in Fig. 7.3, two well-resolved bands were observed in the Raman spectra of the CCY; namely the D band, which is centered at ~1352 cm^{-1} and the G band, which was located at ~1598 cm^{-1}. After dip coated MWCNTs on CCY, The D and G bands were exhibited the same location of CCY with increased intensity [28, 29]. The Raman spectra of Fe_2O_3/MWCNTs/CCY in composite demonstrated five important peaks which the characteristic peaks of hematite standard, namely two A_{1g} mode (223 cm^{-1}, 497 cm^{-1}), and three E_g modes (293 cm^{-1}, 395 cm^{-1} and 615 cm^{-1}) along with carbon peaks [30-32]. These Raman spectral changes of MWCNTs/CCY were due to the anchoring of Fe_2O_3 nanostructures on the MWCNTs/CCY surface. Also, no impurities peaks were identified which ensured the purity of the samples.

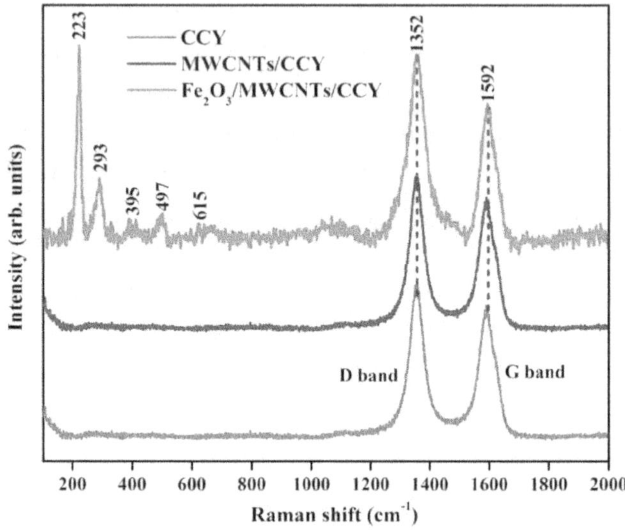

Fig. 7.3 RAMAN spectra of CCY, MWCNTs/CCY and Fe_2O_3/MWCNTs/CCY

The G band is generally related to the in-plane carbon-carbon stretching vibrations of all pairs of sp^2 atoms in the graphite layers; whereas the D band is attributed to the graphite imperfections, arising from the breathing modes of sp^2 atoms in graphitic rings. Furthermore, the crystallinity and graphitization degree of the CCY, MWCNTs/CCY and Fe_2O_3/MWCNTs/CCY were estimated by the peak intensity ratio of the D band and G bands (I_D/I_G value) and the value were found to be 0.65, 1.32 and 1.35 respectively. From these results, it can be seen that the Fe_2O_3/MWCNTs/CCY contain graphitic structures and defects, which may be helpful to enhance the electrochemical performance.

7.3.4 Morphological and compositional analysis of CCY, MWCNTs/CCY and Fe_2O_3/MWCNTs/CCY

Figure 7.4 shows the morphologies of bare CCY, MWCNTs coated CCY and Fe_2O_3 decorated MWCNTs/CCY nanocomposites observed by FESEM. Fig. 7.4a shows the representative FESEM image of carbon yarn. The smooth surface can be observed (Fig. 7.4a, inset) on a single carbon fiber with a diameter of ~ 5 μm. After the dip coating of MWCNTs (Fig. 7.4b), on the rough surface of the carbon fibers can be obtained, indicating the homogeneous and uniform coating of MWCNTs. Fig. 7.4c shows the CCY has been uniformly coated with a smooth thin MWCNTs with the outer and inner diameters of ~15 and ~ 5 nm (Discussed in chapter V).

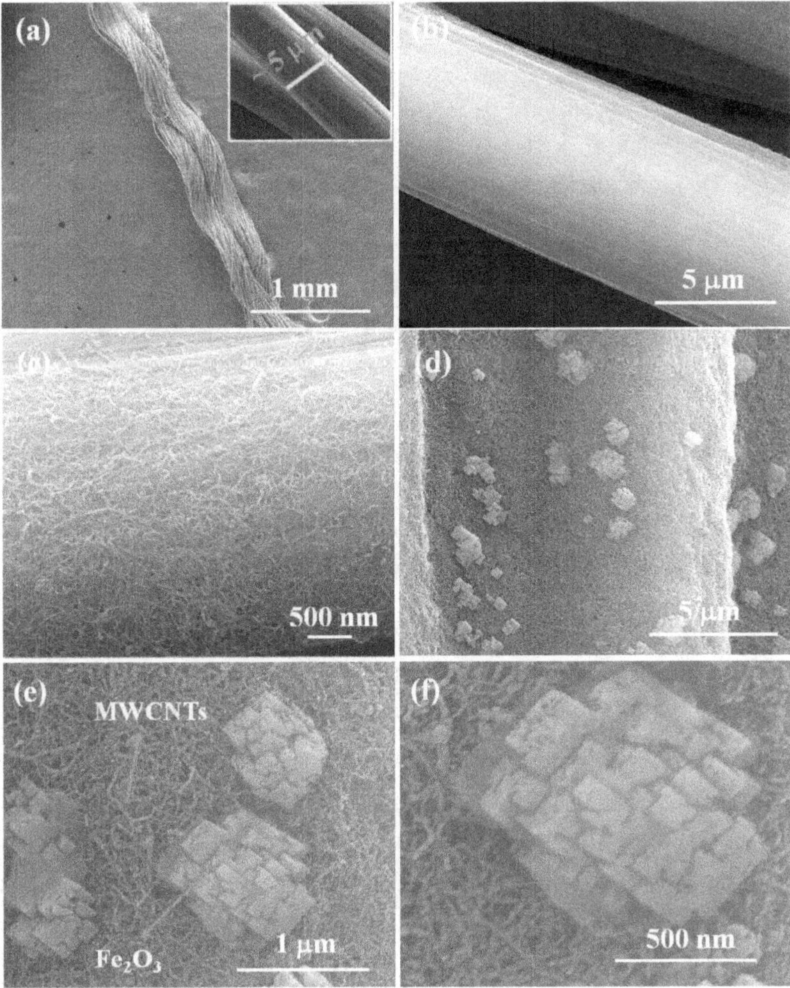

Fig. 7.4 FESEM images of (a) bare CCY, (b & c) MWCNTs/CCY and (d-f) Fe_2O_3/MWCNTs/CCY with different magnifications

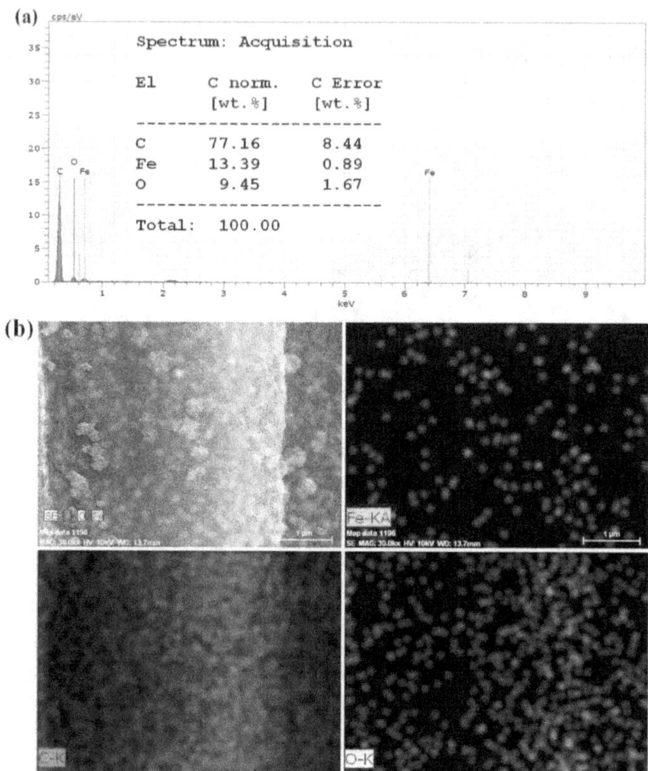

Fig. 7.5 (a) EDS spectra and (b) corresponding FESEM image and EDS mapping of Fe$_2$O$_3$/MWCNTs/CCY

Figure 7.4 d & e shows the uniform deposition of the Fe$_2$O$_3$ nanostructures on the MWCNTs/CCY, the hydrothermal method guaranteed the systematic coating of the Fe$_2$O$_3$ on dip coated MWCNTs/CCY. Fig. 7.4f is the corresponding enlarged view of the Fe$_2$O$_3$ on MWCNTs/CCY, indicating that numerous Fe$_2$O$_3$ nanoparticles uniformly deposited with agglomeration on the surface. The same procedure has been followed for the preparation of Fe$_2$O$_3$ *(Discussed in Chapter IV)* but the morphology of Fe$_2$O$_3$ got distorted. The hydrothermally coated Fe$_2$O$_3$ nanostructure on MWCNTs/CCY can greatly enhance the specific surface area and more active sites to enhance antigen-antibody interactions.

In order to confirm the element composition of the Fe_2O_3 anchored MWCNTs/CCY, the EDS and elemental mapping was obtained which is assigned (Fig. 7.5a) to the elements C, Fe and O, respectively. In EDS results, Carbon percentage showed high which exhibited from the MWCNTs and CCY. Interestingly, the elemental mapping (Fig. 7.5b) of these elements displays a very similar intensity distribution, revealing the effective incorporation and homogeneous distribution of a large quantity of Fe_2O_3 nanostructure throughout the whole structure of MWCNTs dip coated carbon fiber.

7.3.5 Electrical conductivity and mechanical properties of Fe_2O_3/MWCNTs/CCY

The electrical resistance of 5 cm long Fe_2O_3/MWCNTs coated yarn was measured in air by triplet. It has been reported that being a supporting matrix the MWCNTs can enhance the electrical conductivity transition metal oxides [6]. Because of the existence of large amount of MWCNTs/CCY, Fe_2O_3/MWCNTs/CCY exhibited lower resistance than the bare CCY (36 ±1 Ω) and the values found to be 42.5 ±1.5 Ω and 40.2 ±1.1 Ω respectively. Because of the existence of large amount of MWCNTs, Fe_2O_3@MWCNTs exhibited almost equal resistance compare to than the bare CCY. The reasonably low electrical resistance of Fe_2O_3/MWCNTs carbon fiber allows for convenient sensing applications [33]. Also, the conductivity of Fe_2O_3/MWCNTs/CCY was verified by powering an LED device connected to a battery as shown in Fig. 7.6.

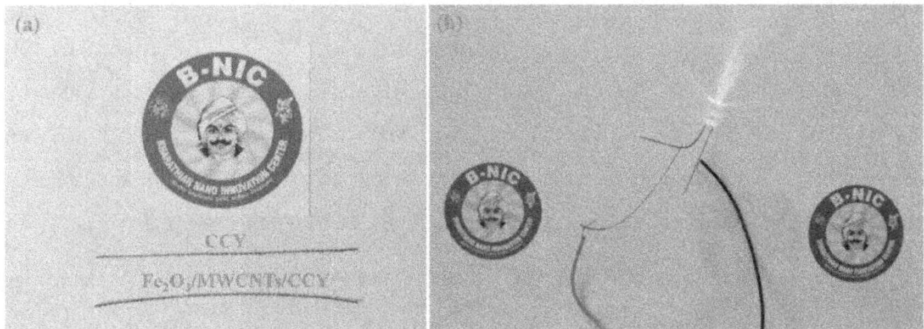

Fig. 7.6 Photographs of Fe_2O_3/MWCNTs/CCY; (a) Comparison of the pure CCY and Fe_2O_3/MWCNTs/CCY and (b) Demonstration of LED emission with the current passing through Fe_2O_3/MWCNTs coated CCY

The mechanical properties of prepared materials were investigated using universal testing machine. The ultimate strength measured for MWCNTs/CCY and Fe_2O_3/MWCNTs/CCY was found to be 40.8±0.8 and 45.3±1 MPa respectively. This value is much higher than the bare CCY (20.10 MPa). This implied that the strength of the yarn got enhanced because of the uniform and intense coating of MWCNTs and Fe_2O_3 on the entire surface of CCY. Also, the elongation and young's modulus of the Fe_2O_3/MWCNTs/CCY (6.82 % and 90.40 MPa) were improved after MWCNTs incorporation (8.87% and 90.4±1.5 MPa). The mechanical strength of the Fe_2O_3/MWCNTs/CCY found higher than that of the pure CCY and MWCNTs/CCY due to a densification, and stronger adhesion of the fibers to each other by the material.

7.3.6 Specific and assessable surface area of CCY, MWCNTs/CCY and Fe_2O_3/MWCNTs/CCY electrode

Specific surface areas were calculated from the results of N_2 physisorption by using the BET analysis. The surface area of the Fe_2O_3/MWCNTs/CCY was identified as 145.32 m^2/g comparable to MWCNTs/CCY (124.32 m^2/g). This outcome of the nanocomposites was clearly indicating, network like interconnected MWCNTS and Fe_2O_3 nanostructures on CCY possessed much higher specific surface area as compared to bare CCY and MWCNTs coated CCY. In order to illustrate that the prepared Fe_2O_3/MWCNTs/CCY nanocomposites could improve the surface area and conductivity of the immunosensor, electroactive surface area (A_e) of bare and modified electrodes was determined by CV using the standard Randles-Sevcik equation [34]. The active surface area was found to be 0.0704 cm^2 for bare CCY, 0.0923 cm^2 for MWCNTs/CCY and 0.0923 cm^2 on Fe_2O_3/MWCNTs/CCY. The active surface area of the nanocomposite electrode can be attributed to the incorporation of Fe_2O_3 nanostructures on MWCNTs/CCY.

7.3.7 Wettability analysis of CCY, MWCNTs/CCY and Fe_2O_3/MWCNTs/CCY electrodes

To disclose a better performance of the Fe_2O_3/MWCNTs/CCY than the MWCNTs/CCY and the bare CCY electrodes, the effect of wettability on wearable electrochemical efficiency were studied and the results displayed in Fig. 7.7.

The wettability was checked by measuring the contact angles of DD water toward the different electrode surfaces Fig.7.7 (inset). After the deposition of MWCNTs on the carbon fibers by dip coating, which were relatively hydrophobic equal to bare CCY. Because, the MWCNT is mostly constituted by hydrophobic carbon atoms with sp^2 hybridization. After the processes of oxidation with acid functionalization, the functional groups introduced onto the side walls caused a change in the contact angle of the water droplet due to hydrogen bonding interactions [35]. Thus, the CNTs deposition has a strong effect on the wettability of carbon fibers in polar liquids. Further, Fe$_2$O$_3$/MWCNTs/CCY surface adsorbing liquid drop with a contact angle of 0°, indicating the superhydrophilic property. It may be the interconnected network structure formed by MWCNTs on fiber surface was beneficial to the spreadability of Fe$_2$O$_3$ nanostructure with improved roughness [36].

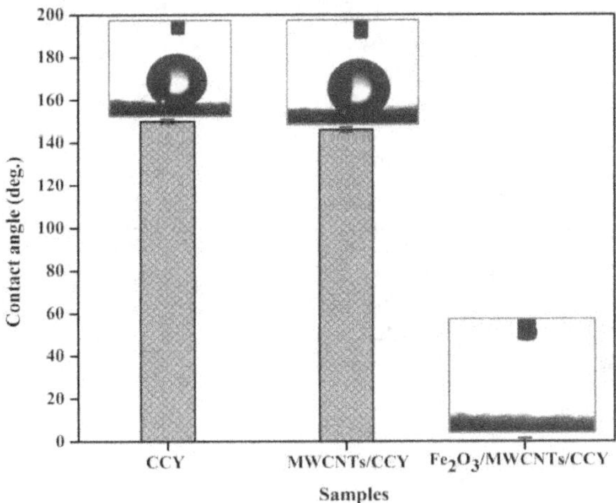

Fig. 7.7 Water contact angle of on CCY, MWCNTs/CCY and Fe$_2$O$_3$/MWCNTs/CCY [Insets: The images of water contact angle]

7.3.8 *In vitro* cell viability evaluation

The cell viability analysis of the prepared Fe$_2$O$_3$/MWCNTs/CCY against fibroblast L929 mouse skin cells was evaluated using the standard MTT assay. The analysis has been done for different concentrations of Fe$_2$O$_3$/MWCNTs/CCY (0.25, 0.5 and 1 mg) as shown in Fig. 7.10. The Fe$_2$O$_3$/MWCNTs/CCY hybrid did not show any significant decrease in cell viability of L929 fibroblast cells even at higher concentration. The corresponding viability results were observed above 97 % for all the three fiber concentrations. Hence, the result indicated the biocompatible characteristic of synthesized Fe_2O_3/MWCNTs/CCY which can be employed as a promising candidate for wearable sensor applications under physiological conditions.

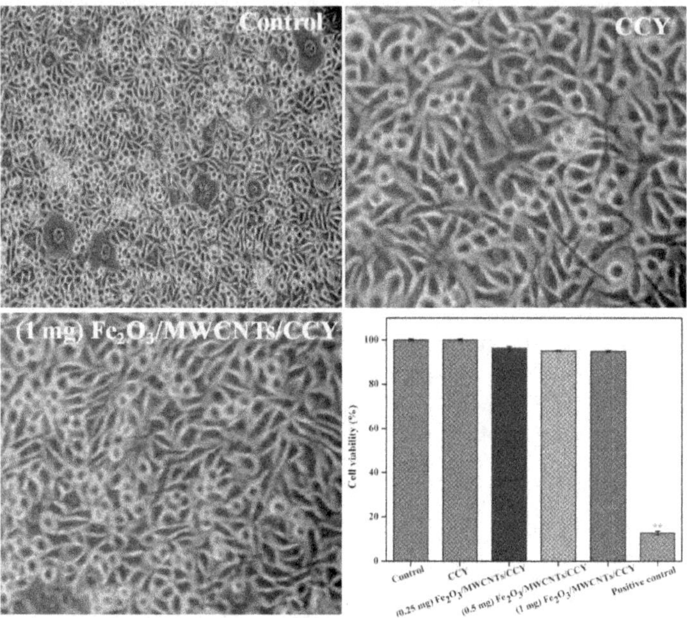

Fig. 7.8 MTT analysis of cultured fibroblast L929 cells treated with different concentration of Fe_2O_3/MWCNTs/CCY samples for 24 hrs. Data represented as mean ± SD of three independent tests. **P<0.01

7.4 Electrochemical analysis

7.4.1 Cyclic voltammetry studies

CV technique was used to optimize the stepwise fabrication of electrochemical immunosensor which was developed to detect cortisol. Fig. 7.9 shows the results of the CV studies for bare CCY, Fe_2O_3/MWCNTs/CCY, Anti-C_{mab}/Fe_2O_3/MWCNTs/CCY and BSA/Anti-C_{mab}/Fe_2O_3/MWCNTs/CCY in 20 mL PBS (pH 7.0) at the scan rate of 50 mV/s in a potential range from − 0.4 to 1.0 V. The CV result of bare CCY showed poor redox response compared to the hybrid. Whereas, Fe_2O_3/MWCNTs/CCY electrode exhibited a well-defined oxidation and reduction peaks corresponding to analyte present in the electrolyte.

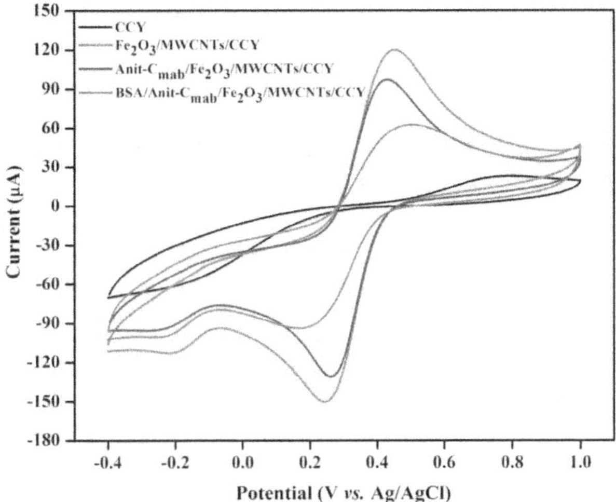

Fig. 7.9 CV analysis of step wise fabrication of BSA/Anti-C_{mab}/Fe_2O_3/MWCNTs/CCY immunoelectrode in PBS (10 mM, pH 7.0)

It can be seen that the magnitude of electrochemical current response decreased after modifying Fe_2O_3/MWCNTs/CCY electrode by EDC/NHS and Anti-C_{mab}. This suggested that Anti-C_{mab} hindered the electron transport due to the successful covalent binding formation between Anti-C_{mab} and EDC/NHS via amide bond formation. The magnitude of current from BSA/Anti-C_{mab}/Fe_2O_3/MWCNTs/CCY immunoelectrode was lower than Anti-C_{mab}/Fe_2O_3/MWCNTs/CCY immunoelectrode. This reduction of current is a clearly indicated that the non-conducting BSA blocks the non-binding sites on immunoelectrode and improved the selectivity of the Fe_2O_3/MWCNTs/CCY electrode.

7.4.2 Effect of pH

CV studies have also been carried out to optimize the suitable pH (PBS solution) for electrochemical measurements. In order to investigate the optimal pH, the activity of BSA/Anti-C_{mab}/Fe_2O_3/MWCNTs/CCY immunoelectrode was investigated in the pH range from 4.5 to 8.5 (Fig. 7.10a). The magnitude of current response was pH dependent and maximum current response was observed at pH 4.5 (Fig. 7.10b). However, it was observed the most stable oxidation and reduction peak area and current response was high for pH 7.0. Further, at pH 7.0 electrolyte behaviors was adjacent to the neutral media, wherein, due to physiological condition electrolyte mimics biological condition. Moreover, the prepared electrodes showed repeatable and reproducible electrochemical response behavior at pH 7.0 and for electrochemical studies which was the recommended pH to get immunocomplex with retained high biological activity [37].

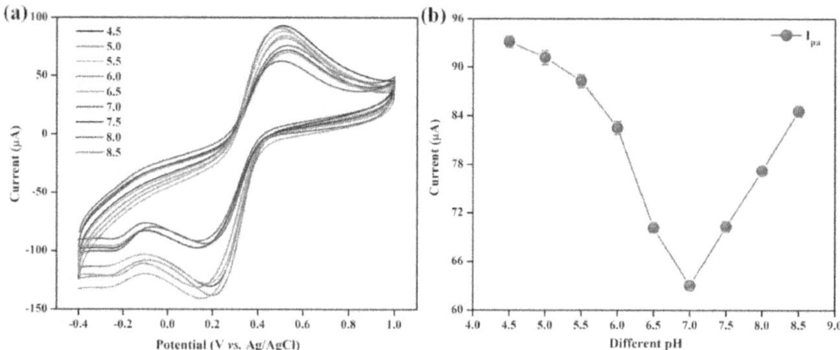

Fig. 7.10 (a) CV analysis of the BSA/Anti-C$_{mab}$/Fe$_2$O$_3$/MWCNTs/CCY immunoelectrode as a function of pH from 4.5 to 8.5 and (b) Linear plots of peak current *vs.* pH values

7.4.3 Effect of scan rate

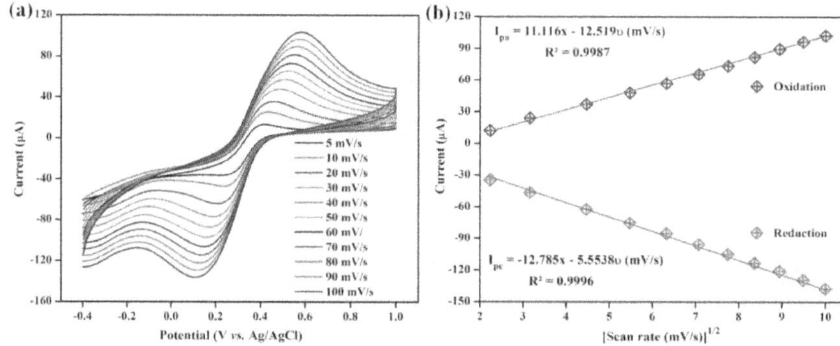

Fig. 7.11 (a) CV analysis of the BSA/Anti-C$_{mab}$/Fe$_2$O$_3$/MWCNTs/CCY immunoelectrode as a function of scan rates (5 to 100 mV/s) in PBS (10 mM, pH 7.0) and (b) Linear plot of the oxidation and reduction peak currents *vs.* square root of scan rates

The scan rate having the greater influence in kinetics of electrochemical reaction, the CV studies of BSA/Anti-C$_{mab}$/Fe$_2$O$_3$/MWCNTs/CCY (Fig. 7.11a) were carried out as a function of scan rate (5–100 mV/s). The magnitude of electrochemical current response and potential of the electrode was found linearly dependent to square root of scan rate and current response as displayed in Fig. 7.11b. The observed well-defined stable redox peaks as a function of scan rate suggested that it was a surface-controlled electrochemical process and diffusion of electrons on surface is taking place in a controlled manner.

The corresponding linear equations are given in *Eq.* 7.1 & 7.2,

$$I_{pa}(\mu A) = 11.116x - 12.519\upsilon\ (mV/s);\ R^2 = 0.9987 \ ----- (Eq.7.1)$$

$$I_{pc}(\mu A) = -12.785 - 5.5538\upsilon\ (mV/s);\ R^2 = 0.9996 \ ------ (Eq.7.2)$$

7.4.4 Cortisol response studies of BSA/Anti-C$_{mab}$/Fe$_2$O$_3$/MWCNTs/CCY immunoelectrode by CV

The electrochemical response of BSA/Anti-C$_{mab}$/Fe$_2$O$_3$/MWCNTs/CCY immunoelectrode (Fig. 7.12a) has been studied as a function of cortisol concentration (1 fg -1 µg) using CV technique under identical experimental conditions of PBS (10 mM, pH 7.0). It is can be seen from Fig. 7.12a that the electrochemical response current decreased with increasing cortisol concentration (1 fg -1 µg). This is due to the formation of immuno complexes between Anti-C$_{mab}$ and cortisol was resulting in electron charge transfer hindrance at the electrode electrolyte interface. The magnitude of electrochemical response current of BSA/Anti-C$_{mab}$/Fe$_2$O$_3$/MWCNTs/CCY immunoelectrode was linearly dependent to the logarithm of cortisol concentration (Fig. 7.12b) and obeyed the following linear equation of Eq. 7.3.

$$\Delta I\ (\mu A) = -0.9591x + 49.546\ [Cortisol\ conc.(g/mL);\ R^2 = 0.9992 \ --(Eq.7.3)$$

The prepared BSA/Anti-C$_{mab}$/Fe$_2$O$_3$/MWCNTs/CCY immunoelectrode exhibited linear range from 1 fg -1 µg and a detection limit of 2.6 fg/mL with a correlation coefficient of 0.9992 which was calculated using the equation of 2.3.

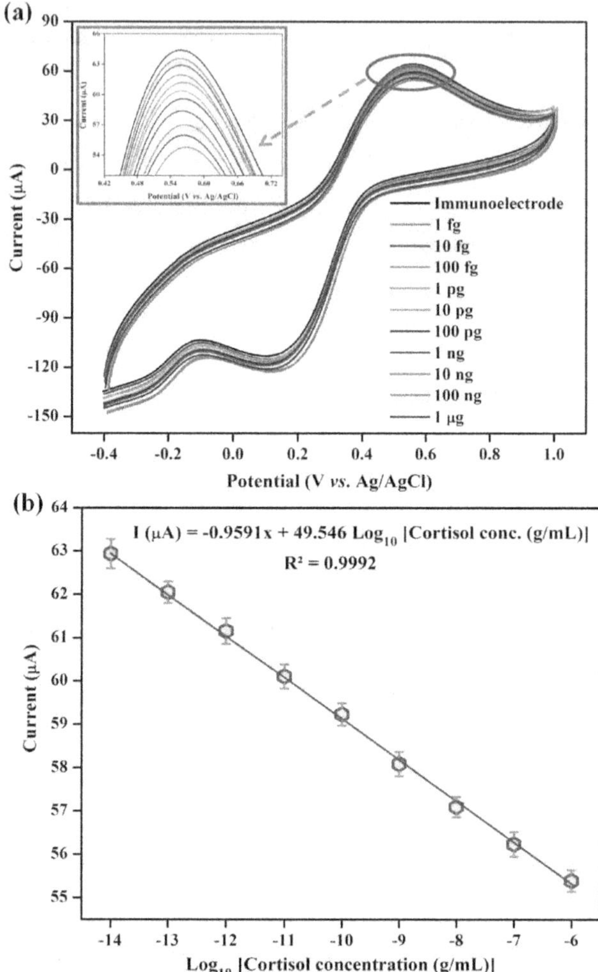

Fig. 7.12 (a) Electrochemical studies of BSA/Anti-C_{mab}/Fe_2O_3/MWCNTs/CCY immunoelectrode as a function of cortisol concentration varied from 10 fg to 1 µg in PBS (10 mM, pH 7.0) and (b) Linear plot between electrochemical peak current response and logarithm of cortisol concentration

7.4.5 Cortisol response studies of BSA/Anti-C$_{mab}$/Fe$_2$O$_3$/MWCNTs/CCY immunoelectrode by DPV

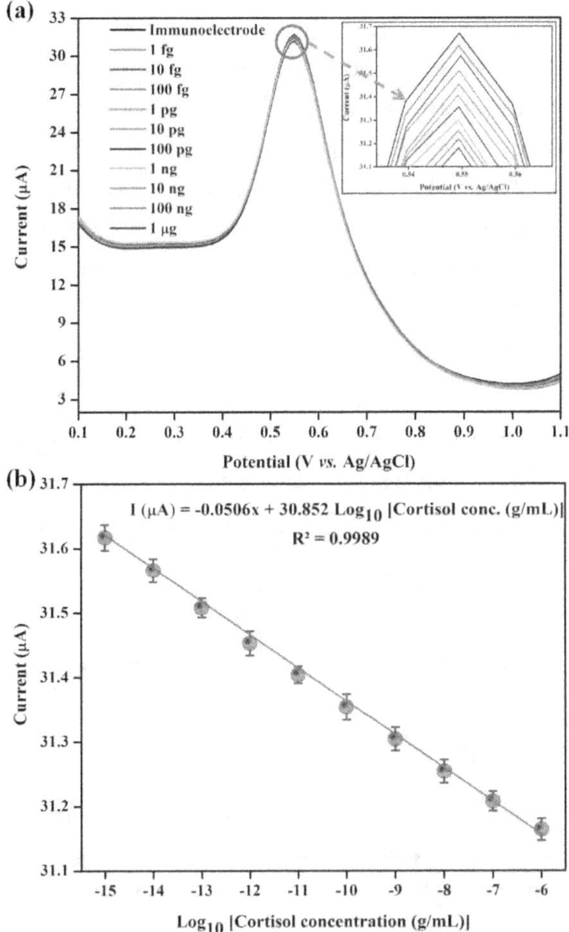

Fig. 7.13 (a) DPV analysis of the BSA/Anti-Cmab/Fe2O3/MWCNTs/CCY immunoelectrode as a function of cortisol concentration varied from 1 fg to 1 µg in PBS (10 mM, pH 7.0) and (b) Linear plot between electrochemical peak current response and logarithm of cortisol concentration

The electrochemical response of the BSA/Anti-C_{mab}/Fe$_2$O$_3$/MWCNTs/CCY immunoelectrode has been studied as a function of cortisol concentration (Fig. 7.13) using the sensitive DPV technique in PBS (10 mM, pH 7.0). DPV is a sensitive analytical technique to study electrochemical changes during biological reactions on the surface, mainly for signal amplification when the analyte concentration is very low [38]. All the measurements for cortisol detection at different concentrations were repeated thrice using different electrodes. During the response study, the magnitude of the electrochemical response current of the BSA/Anti-C_{mab}/Fe$_2$O$_3$/MWCNTs/CCY immunoelectrode was observed to decrease on increasing the cortisol concentration (Fig. 7.13a). This confirmed the successful formation of an immuno-complex between the antigen and the antibody. These results evident the hindrances in electron transfer to the electrode due to the insulating behavior of cortisol.

A linear calibration curve (Fig. 7.13b) obtained between the logarithm of cortisol concentration and the magnitude of electrochemical response current revealed good linear range from 1 fg - 1 µg and followed the linear equation (*Eq.* 7.4),

$$\Delta I\ (\mu A) = -0.0506x + 30.852\ [Cortisol\ conc.\ (g/mL);\ R^2 = 0.9989\ --(Eq.\,7.4)$$

The prepared immunosensor showed excellent response at low concentration of analyte from 1 fg/mL to upper limit of 1 µg/mL with a correlation coefficient of 0.9989. Also, the detection limit of the fabricated immunosensor has been estimated as 0.18 fg/mL using the formula *Eq.* 2.3.

7.4.6 Interference studies

BSA/Anti-Cmab/Fe2O3/MWCNTs/CCY immunoelectrode have been tested for its selectivity among the cortisol analogues (100 ng/mL) namely progesterone, testosterone, corticosterone, cortisone, cholesterol and BSA in presence of cortisol (100 ng/mL) using the DPV technique in PBS (10 mM, pH 7.0) and the results were given in (Fig. 7.14).

The prepared immunosensor showed the current responses after the simultaneous addition of interferents species from the 100 ng/mL cortisol and no significant difference was found. The change in electrochemical response of the interferents was compared to that of the immunosensor and it was found to be of the order of 1–2%. The tests were conducted in triplicate by the standard addition method. This demonstrated that the effect of interferents on BSA/Anti-Cmab/Fe2O3/MWCNTs/CCY immunosensor was negligible and the electrode was found to be very selective to the stress biomarker.

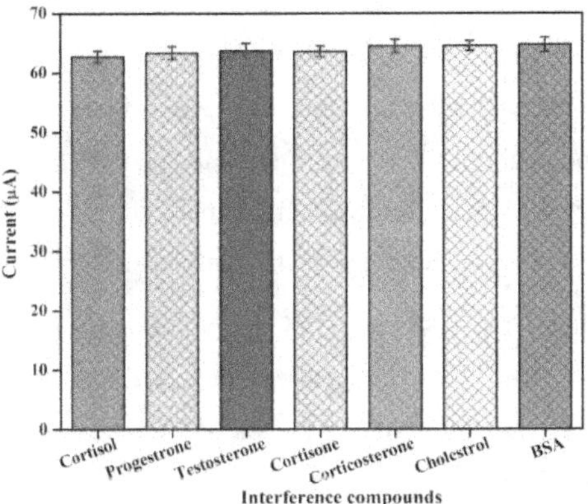

Fig. 7.14 Interference studies of BSA/Anti-C$_{mab}$/Fe$_2$O$_3$/MWCNTs/CCY immunoelectrode towards Progesterone, Testosterone, Cortisone, Corticosterone, Cholesterol and BSA with respect to cortisol (100 ng/mL) in PBS (10 mM, pH 7.0)

7.4.7 Stability, repeatability and reproducibility studies

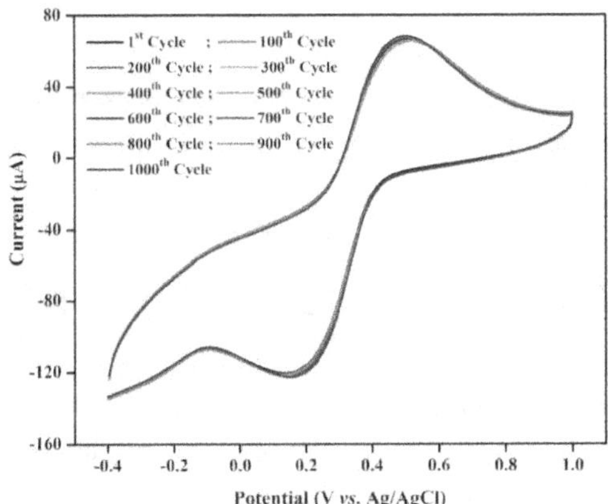

Fig. 7.15 The stability analysis of Fe$_2$O$_3$/MWCNTs/CCY immunoelectrode for 1000 cycles in 10 mM PBS

The stability of Fe_2O_3/MWCNTs/CCY was investigated by measuring the current response using CV method for 1000 cycles in 10 mM PBS as shown in Fig. 7.15. The RSD values were calculated from the current responses obtained for Fe_2O_3/MWCNTs/CCY of 3.08 % which indicating the good stability the modified fiber. The good stability of the immunosensor attributed from the strong interactions between the Fe_2O_3/MWCNTs and cortisol. The slow decrease in response might be due to the gradual deactivation of the immobilized target molecule. Additionally, the immunosensor was stored at 4 °C for four weeks and then it used to detect cortisol in samples, the immunosensor still retained 96.16% of its response which ensured the stability of the electrode.

The RSD value of 3.8 % was found for 10 measurements of 100 ng/mL of cortisol by single binder free BSA/Anti-C_{mab}/Fe_2O_3/MWCNTs/CCY immunoelectrode which revealed the repeatability of developed immunosensor. The five BSA/Anti-C_{mab}/Fe_2O_3/MWCNTs/CCY immunoelectrodes were prepared and evaluated the inter-assay precision or the reproducibility of this modified electrode by measuring cortisol level (100 ng/mL). The average RSD of the intra-and inter-assay was 4.15%, at the cortisol concentration. Thus, these results indicated the fabricated immunosensor has acceptable stability repeatability and reproducibility.

7.4.8 Real sample analysis

We further inspected the possibility of applying the prepared binder free BSA/Anti-C_{mab}/Fe_2O_3/MWCNTs/CCY immunosensor in clinical systems via analyzing several collected real sweat samples and the results were compared with the commercially available CLIA method. Table 7.1 shows the correlation results obtained using the proposed immunosensor and the CILA method (Fig. 7.16).

The RSD values were obtained in the range of 3.245 - 5.215 % and the recovery rates of the samples ranged between 98.01 and 102.542 %. This result obviously elicited that there was no significant difference was observed between the electrochemical and CILA outcomes. Based on the good accuracy and reliability of the proposed method, it could be reasonably applied in the clinical determination of cortisol in human sweat.

Table 7.1 Comparison of sweat cortisol estimated using chemiluminescence immunoassay and Fe_2O_3/MWCNTs/CCY based electrochemical immunosensor

Samples	CLIA method (ng/mL)	Fe_2O_3/MWCNTs/CCY immunosensor				
		Measured (ng/mL)*	Added (ng/mL)	Found (ng/mL)*	RSD (%)	Recovery (%)
1	32	32.89	50	81.25	4.584	98.012
2	49	50.63	50	100.02	3.754	99.393
3	43	42.56	50	91.26	3.245	102.542
4.	51	52.45	50	101.92	5.215	99.482
5.	78	78.98	50	127.85	4.574	99.123

*** The average value of three successive experiments.**

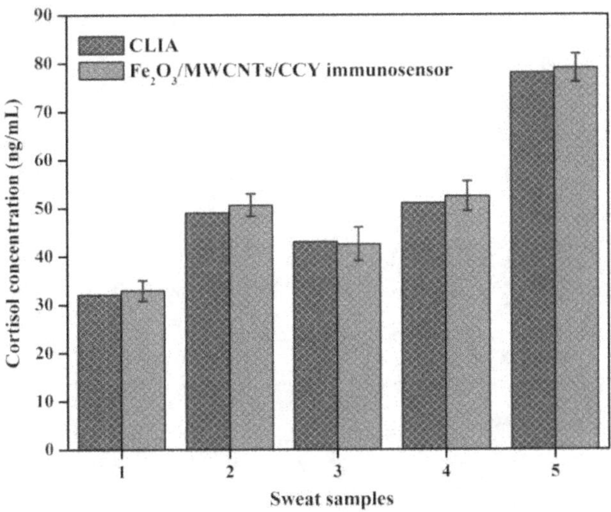

Fig. 7.16 Comparison graph of sweat cortisol estimated using chemiluminescence immunoassay and Fe_2O_3/MWCNTs/CCY based electrochemical immunosensor

7.5 Conclusions

In this chapter, the development of a simple competitive binder free electrochemical immunosensor based Fe_2O_3/MWCNTs/CCY hybrid electrode for the detection of cortisol in human sweat is reported. For this, α-Fe_2O_3 nanoparticles have been successfully embedded on MWCNTs coated CCY back bone to make a highly electro-active Fe_2O_3/MWCNTs/CCY nanocomposite using simple hydrothermal method. Crystallinity, structure, morphology, flexibility, surface area, and elemental analysis were studied by using conventional analytical techniques. The immunosensing approach endorsed the role of immobilization and revealed the significance of covalently immobilized cortisol monoclonal antibody in cortisol sensing. The downside of the MWCNTs in surface wettability was arrested with aid of embedded Fe_2O_3. Hence, the fabricated sensor exhibited an excellent analytical performance in circumstances of sensitivity, selectivity and wider linear range of quantifiable analyte concentrations due to the combinational benefits of the constituents of the hybrids. Further optimization in the composition of the hybrid would offer a practical and affordable analytical tool for the rapid determination of cortisol in clinical applications.

References

1. K. Haghi, O. S. Oluwafemi, J. P. Jose, H. J. Maria, Composites and nanocomposites, 1st Edition, *Publisher: Apple Academic Press*, **(2013)** *ISBN-978-1926895284.*

2. S. Iijima, Helical microtubules of graphitic carbon, *Nature,* **354** (1991) 56–58.

3. G. G. Wildgoose, C. E. Banks, R. G. Compton, Metal Nanoparticles and Related Materials Supported on Carbon Nanotubes: Methods and Applications, *Small,* **2** (2006) 182-193.

4. P. J. F. Harris, Carbon nanotube composites, *Int. Mater. Rev.,* **49** (2004) 31-43.

5. H. C. Zeng, In Handbook of Organic-Inorganic Hybrid Materials and Nanocomposites, *Publishers: American Scientific,* Stevenson Ranch, (2003), *Nanocomposites,* **Chapter 4,** 151-180.

6. N. Yan, X. Zhou , Y. Li, F. Wang, H. Zhong, H. Wang, Q. Chen, Fe_2O_3 Nanoparticles Wrapped in multi-walled carbon nanotubes with enhanced lithium storage capability, *Sci. Rep.,* **3** (2013) 3392 (1-6).

7. B. Xue, P. Chen, Q. Hong, J. Lin, K. L. Tan, Growth of Pd, Pt, Ag and Au nanoparticles on carbon nanotubes, *J. Mater. Chem.,* **11** (2001) 2378-2381.

8. Y. T. Kim, K. Ohshima, K. Higashimine, T. Uruga, M. Takata, H. Suematsu, T. Mitani, Fine size control of platinum on carbon nanotubes: from single atoms to clusters, *Angew. Chem., Int. Ed.* **45** (2006) 407-411.

9. S. Banerjee and S. S. Wong, Synthesis and Characterization of Carbon Nanotube−Nanocrystal Heterostructures, *Nano Lett.,* **2** (2002) 195-200.

10. J. Sun, L. Gao, M. Iwasa, Noncovalent attachment of oxide nanoparticles onto carbon nanotubes using water-in-oil microemulsions, *Chem. Commun.,* **0** (2004) 832-833.

11. J. Du, L. Fu, Z. Liu, B. Han, Z. Li, Y. Liu, Z. Sun, D. Zhu, Facile route to synthesize multiwalled carbon nanotube/zinc sulfide heterostructures: optical and electrical properties, *J. Phys. Chem. B,* **109** (2005) 12772-12776.

12. J. Li, S. Tang, L. Lu, H. C. Zeng, Preparation of nanocomposites of metals, metal oxides, and carbon nanotubes via self-assembly, *J. Am. Chem. Soc.,* **129** (2007) 9401-9409.

13. X. Chen, Z. Zhao, Y. Zhou, Y. Shu, M. Sajjad, Q. Bi, Y. Ren, X. Wang, X. Zhou, Z. Liu, MWCNTs modified α-Fe_2O_3 nanoparticles as anode active materials and carbon nanofiber paper as a flexible current collector for lithium-ion batteries application, *J Alloys Compd.,* **776** (2019) 974-983.

14. X. R. Lin, Y. F. Zheng, X. C. Song, Fe_2O_3/MWCNTs nanocomposite decorated glassy carbon electrode for the determination of nitrite, *Bull. Mater. Sci.,* **41** (2018) 35 (1-7)

15. B. Sun, Y. Gou, Yu. Ma, X. Zheng, R. Bai, A. Attia, A. Abdelmoaty, F. Hu, Investigate electrochemical immunosensor of cortisol based on gold nanoparticles/ magnetic functionalized reduced graphene oxide, *Biosens. Bioelectron,* **88** (2017) 55-62.

16. T. T. Yu, H. L. Liu, M. Huang, J. H. Zhang, D. Q. Su, Z. H. Tang, J. F. Xie, Y. J. Liu, A. H. Yuan, Q. H. Kong, Zn_2GeO_4 nanorods grown on carbon cloth as high performance flexible lithium-ion battery anodes, *RSC Adv.,* **7** (2017) 51807–51813.

17. Y. Li, C. Tian, W. Liu, S. Xu, Y. Xu, R. Cui, Z. Lin, Carbon Cloth Supported Nano-$Mg(OH)_2$ for the Enrichment and Recovery of Rare Earth Element Eu(III) From Aqueous Solution, *Front Chem.,* **6** (2018) 1-9.

18. D. Maity, K. Rajavel, R. T. Rajendrakumar, Polyvinyl alcohol wrapped multiwall carbon nanotube (MWCNTs) network on fabrics for wearable room temperature ethanol sensor, *Sens. Actuator B-Chem.,* **261** (2018) 297-306.

19. X. Wu, H. Xie, Q. Deng, H. X. Wang, H. Sheng, Y.X. Yin, W. X. Zhou, R.L. Li, Yu-G. Guo, Three-dimensional carbon nanotubes forest/carbon cloth as an efficient electrode for Li-polysulfide batteries, *ACS Appl. Mater. Interfaces,* **18** (2017) 1553-1561.

20. N. Yan, X. Zhou, Y. Li, F. Wang, H. Zhong, H. Wang, Q. Chen, Fe_2O_3 nanoparticles wrapped in multi-walled carbon nanotubes with enhanced lithium storage capability, *Sci. Rep.,* **3** (2013) 3392 (1-6).

21. S. S. Raut and B. R. Sankapal, Comparative studies on MWCNTs, Fe_2O_3 and Fe_2O_3/MWCNTs thin films towards supercapacitor application, *New J. Chem.,* **40** (2016) 2619-2627.

22. K. G. Chandrappa and T. V. Venkatesha, Electrochemical bulk synthesis of Fe_3O_4 and a-Fe_2O_3 nanoparticles and its Zn–Co–a–Fe_2O_3 composite thin films for corrosion protection, *Materials and Corrosion*, **63** (2012) 1-13.

23. D. Hirayama, C. Saron, E. C. Botelho, M. L. Costac, A. C. Ancelotti, Polypropylene composites manufactured from recycled carbon fibers from aeronautic materials waste, *Mater. Res.*, **20** (2017) 519-525.

24. J. Song, Q. Yuan, X. Liu, D. Wang, F. Fu, W. Yang, Combination of nitrogen plasma modification and waterborne polyurethane treatment of carbon fiber paper used for electric heating of wood floors, *BioResources*, **10** (2015) 5820-5829.

25. V. Eswaraiah, V. Sankaranarayanan, S. Ramaprabhu, Inorganic nanotubes reinforced polyvinylidene fluoride composites as low-cost electromagnetic interference shielding materials, *Nanoscale Res. Lett.*, **37** (2011) 1-12.

26. M. A. Karimiama, F. Banifatemeh, A. H. Mehrjardi, H. Tavallali, G. D. Rad, A novel rapid synthesis of Fe_2O_3/grapheme nanocomposite using ferrate(VI) and its application as a new kind of nanocomposite modified electrode as electrochemical sensor, *Mater Res Bull.*, **70** (2015) 856-864.

27. A. Rufus, N. Sreej, D. Philip, Synthesis of biogenic hematite (α-Fe_2O_3) nanoparticles for antibacterial and nanofluid applications, *RSC Adv.*, **6** (2016) 94206-94217.

28. J. Guo, C. Lu, F. An, Effect of electrophoretically deposited carbon nanotubes on the interface of carbon fiber reinforced epoxy composite, *J Mater Sci.*, **47** (2012) 2831–2836.

29. S. Luo, Y. Wang, G. Wang, K. Wang, Z. Wang, C. Zhang, B. Wang, Y. Luo, L. Li, T. Liu, CNT Enabled Co-braided smart fabrics: A new route for noninvasive, highly sensitive & large area monitoring of composites, *Sci. Rep.*, **7** (2017) 44056 (1-10).

30. T. Szatkowski, M. Wysokowski, G. Lota, D. Peziak, V. V. Bazhenov, G. Nowaczyk, J. Walter, S. L. Molodtsov, H. Stocker, C. Himcinschi, I. Petrenko, A. L. Stelling, S. Jurga, D. T. Jesionowski, H. Ehrlich, *RSC Adv.*, **5** (2015) 79031–79040.

31. E. M. Verdugo, Y. Xie, J. Baltrusaitisc, D. M. Cwiertny, Hematite decorated multi-walled carbon nanotubes (α-Fe_2O_3/MWCNTs) as sorbents for Cu(II) and Cr(VI): comparison of hybrid sorbent performance to its nanomaterial building blocks, *RSC Adv.*, **6** (2016) 99997–100007.

32. D. L. A. S. de Faria, S.V. Silva, M. T. de Oliveira, Raman Microspectroscopy of Some Iron Oxides and Oxyhydroxides, *J. Raman Spectrosc.*, **28** (1997) 873-878.

33. B. S. Shim, W. Chen, C. Doty, C. Xu, N. A. Kotov, Smart electronic yarns and wearable fabrics for human biomonitoring made by carbon nanotube coating with polyelectrolytes, *Nano Lett.*, **8** (2008) 4151-4157.

34. H.T. Purushothama, Y. Arthoba Nayaka, Electrochemical study of hydrochlorothiazide on electrochemically pretreated pencil graphite electrode as a sensor, *Sens Biosensing Res.*, **16** (2017) 12–18.

35. J. Guo, C. Lu, F. An, Effect of electrophoretically deposited carbon nanotubes on the interface of carbon fiber reinforced epoxy composite, *J Mater Sci.*, **47** (2012) 2831–2836.

36. C. Lyu, J. Zheng, R. Zhang, R. Zou, B. Liu, W. Zhou, Homologous Co_3O_4‖CoP nanowires grown on carbon cloth as a high-performance electrode pair for triclosan degradation and hydrogen evolution, *Mater. Chem. Front.*, **2** (2018) 323-330.

37. A. Vasudeva, A. Kaushik, Y. Tomizawa, N. Norena, S. Bhansali, An LTCC-based microfluidic system for label-free, electrochemical detection of cortisol, *Sens. Actuator B-Chem.*, **182** (2013) 139– 146.

38. R. Sriramprabha, M. Divagar, D. Mangalaraj, N. Ponpandian, C. Viswanathan, Formulation of SnO_2/graphene nanocomposite modified electrode for synergetic electrochemical detection of dopamine, *Adv. Mater. Lett.*, **6** (2015) 973-977.

Chapter VIII

The modern lifestyle of today's world suffered serious life-threatening diseases like heart disease, mental problems and depression which have become major issue in developing countries. Due to these problems, rate of psychological stress is increasing alarmingly. Psychological stress affects the nervous system and health due to the in cortisol level. The commercial cortisol detection techniques using various bio-fluids, in which sweat is the most extensively evaluated non-invasive body fluid as it contains plethora of medical information for diagnosis in POC. This inevitable factor motivated us to develop metal oxides like SnO_2, TiO_2, Fe_2O_3 and ZnO with desired morphologies along with MWCNTs based hybrid materials on CCY, which is a new area for developing the sensor platforms employed in wearable sensors.

The present work described the preparation and evaluation of immunosensing performance of the developed electrodes and the overall results are summarized (Table 8.1) and discussed as follows.

In general, the sensor electrodes are expected to have high surface area, fast charge transfer ability, preferred wettability in aqueous solution along with better mechanical stability. The prepared metal oxides belong to different crystal systems with the average crystalline size in the range of 6-12 nm. The smaller sized crystal could have higher surface area. The calculated specific and active surface area values from BET and electrochemical analysis evidenced the effective sensing proficiency of the prepared electrodes. In particular Fe_2O_3 integrated CCY exhibited higher surface area compared to other prepared electrodes.

The reasonable hardness and elastic modulus values of the fiber based electrodes assured their mechanical stability and the conductivity measurements also endorsed their charge transfer ability. The wettability study also aided the applicability of the prepared electrodes for sweat based sensor applications. Though all the physico-chemical results demonstrated the sensing ability of the prepared electrodes, comparably Fe_2O_3 integrated CCY revealed better sensor perspectives which may be resulted from its morphology and surface features.

Table 8.1 Summary of present work outcomes

Immuno electrodes	Structural characterizations							Electrochemical characterizations						
	Crystal system/ Grain Size	Morph ology	Resistance (Ω)	Hardness/ Young's modulus (MPa)	Specific surface area (m^2/g)	Active Surface area (cm^2)	Contact angle ($°$)	CV		DPV		Stability (%)	Real Sample analysis	
								Linear range	LOD	Linear range	LOD		RSD range (%)	Recovery (%)
SnO$_2$/CCY	Tetragonal/ ~ 6 nm	Nano flakes	68±1.5	31.86 /48.34	115.12	0.0852	47.1	1 pg to 1 µg	4.5 pg	10 fg to 1 µg	1.6 fg	95.40	2.28 - 4.25	99.02 - 102.93
TiO$_2$/CCY	Tetragonal/ ~ 6 nm	Nano cubes	63.4±1.8	28.46/ 42.56	108.48	0.0894	0	10 fg to 1 µg	17 fg	10 fg to 1 µg	6.16 fg	94.70	3.06 - 5.83	96.01 - 104.60
Fe$_2$O$_3$/CCY	Rhombohedral/ ~ 12 nm	Nano ellipsoid	58±1.2	**33.27/ 67.03**	**146.02**	**0.0942**	**0**	1 fg to 1 µg	0.005 fg	1 fg to 1 µg	0.003	95.28	3.40 - 4.06	98.67 - 104.2
ZnO NRs/CCY	Hexagonal ~ 12 nm	Nanorods	54.3±1.2	38.40/ 57.17	138.116	0.0932	0	1 fg to 1 µg	0.45 fg	1 fg to 1 µg	0.98 fg	96.23	2.33 - 4.46	97.95 - 103.36
MWCNTs/ CCY	Amorphous carbon	Nanotubes	42.55±1	40.82/ 82.74	122.54	0.0858	150	10 fg to 1 µg	2.69 fg	10 fg to 1 µg	0.56 fg	95.20	3.25 - 5.13	95.46 - 104.73
Fe$_2$O$_3$/ MWCNTs /CCY	Rhombohedral- amorphous carbon	Nanotubes	40.2 ±1.1	45.30/ 90.40	145.32	0.0923	0	1 fg to 1 µg	2.6 fg	1 fg to 1 µg	0.18 fg	96.16	3.25 - 5.22	98.01 - 102.54

Despite the same immobilization protocol has been followed to transfer cortisol antibodies on the all fiber electrodes, the electrochemical responses from CV analysis in pH 7.0 of Fe_2O_3 and its composite based immunoelectrodes only showed minimum current response which assured the high enzyme loading capacity. The scan rate results illustrated the electrochemical kinetics of the all prepared immunoelectrodes was surface controlled quasi-reversible process.

The linear detection range and limit of detection values determined for the developed immunoelectrodes were lying in the range of 1 fg to 1 µg and the ultra sensitive ability was identified for Fe_2O_3, ZnO and MWCNTs based sensor platforms. Finally the cortisol quantification in human sweat sample and validation results from CILA method also proved that the practical applicability of the developed immunosensor in real time applications.

Therefore fruitful outcomes of the present work can be served as an affordable analytical tool for the rapid determination of cortisol in clinical and POC applications for developing smart textiles.

Scope of the future work

- Optimization of carbon and polymer based hybrids for effective cortisol sensing.

- Other cross-linkers can be tested to scrutinize for the effective antibody immobilization

- A detailed biocompatibility analysis in skill cell lines have to be carried out for the developed hybrid electrodes used in wearable sensors

- The sweat absorbing area will be developed in order to make it usable for smart textile applications.